PREFACE

This handbook is in its fourth edition and is dealing with the difficult assignment of informing the scientific community of the pathophysiology and management of pain. The management of pain is one of the most demanding tasks that faces the medical community. Since one of the major problems is the understanding of the wide variety of pharmacologic and non-pharmacologic approached to pain management, the **HANDBOOK OF PAIN MANAGEMENT, Fourth Edition**, addresses not only the pharmacology of various therapeutic agents useful in the treatment of pain, but also a number of non-pharmacologic treatment modalities.

The handbook is divided into the following areas: (1) Pathophysiology and Biochemistry of Pain, (2) Pharmacology of Analgesic Drugs, (3) Management of Pain, (4) Selected Drug Interactions, (5) an explanation of the Controlled Substances Act, and (6) Miscellaneous Drug Tables. The *Pathophysiology* section provides a brief, but concise description of the anatomy of neural pain pathways and biochemistry involved in pain mechanisms. Detailed descriptions of the pain pathways are presented along with information on the neurotransmitters which have been implicated in pain. The *Pharmacology* section deals with the pharmacology of the analgesics and presents the classification, mechanisms of action, therapeutic and adverse effects on various organ systems, pharmacokinetics, and individual drug monographs on both the opioid (narcotic) and non-opioid (nonsteroidal anti-inflammatory) analgesic compounds. The section on *Management of Pain* is designed to provide an overview of basic therapeutic approaches to both acute and chronic pain patients, including a discussion on the psychological considerations in the management of chronic pain. There is also information on the treatment three common clinical situations in which pain may be problematic: rheumatoid arthritis, low back pain, and trigeminal neuralgia. A few drug interactions have been chosen and are outlined in the *Selected Drug Interactions* section and there is a short discussion of the *Controlled Substances Act*. The *Miscellaneous Drug Tables* section contains tables of single opioid and non-opioid analgesic preparations, combination products that are available, analgesic adjuvants, and the common adult and pediatric dosages of these drugs. In addition this section contains a variety of other tables that are useful to practicing physicians who deal with patients in pain.

Based on our past experiences, we believe that the entire medical community (including practicing physicians, medical residents and interns, nurses, physician assistants, pharmacists, medical students, and researchers) who have an interest in dealing with patients in pain will benefit from the material contained within.

The Authors

Handbook of Pain Management

Fourth Edition

G. John DiGregorio, M.D., Ph.D.
Professor of Pharmacology and Medicine
Hahnemann University School of Medicine
Philadelphia, Pennsylvania

Edward J. Barbieri, Ph.D.
Associate Professor of Pharmacology
Hahnemann University School of Medicine
Philadelphia, Pennsylvania

Andrew P. Ferko, Ph.D.
Associate Professor of Pharmacology
Hahnemann University School of Medicine
Philadelphia, Pennsylvania

Gerald H. Sterling, Ph.D.
Associate Professor of Pharmacology
Temple University School of Medicine
Philadelphia, Pennsylvania

John F. Camp, M.D.
Clinical Assistant Professor in Anesthesiology
University of North Carolina Medical School
Chapel Hill, North Carolina

Maurice F. Prout, Ph.D.
Assistant Professor
Institute for Graduate Clinical Psychology
Widener University
Chester, Pennsylvania

1994

HANDBOOK OF PAIN MANAGEMANT

Fourth Edition

Printed in the United States of America.

TABLE OF CONTENTS

PAGE

PAGE

PAGE

PATHOPHYSIOLOGY

AND

BIOCHEMISTRY

OF

PAIN

INTRODUCTION

The management of pain is probably one of the commonest and yet most difficult aspects of medical practice, despite the large number of effective analgesic agents available for clinical use and an understanding of the mechanisms by which they are effective. Most acute pain situations, those that arise from an acute injury or disease and have a limited duration, are usually easily treated. It is the more chronic pain syndromes that challenge the therapeutic skills of the physician. This is complicated by the subjective nature of pain and its tendency to be influenced by the behavioral state of the patient. Furthermore, drugs that reduce or alleviate pain may cause dependence, addiction and iatrogenic disease on long term use. In order to derive an appropriate therapeutic approach to pain, the physician must have an intimate understanding of the anatomy, biochemistry and pathophysiology associated with pain and of the various classes of analgesic drugs and their characteristics, including potency against a particular type of pain, pharmacokinetic properties and the potential for addiction and toxicity.

Pain is the most immediate, direct and compelling of sensations. When a patient experiences pain, he/she comes to the physician with expectations of immediate relief. Pain can be defined as a sensory experience evoked by stimuli that injure or threaten to destroy tissue, e.g., the pain of angina due to myocardial ischemia. This definition of pain, involving some tissue pathology, fits well with the description and appropriate treatment of acute pain. However, there are many chronic pain situations in which no tissue pathology can be found, e.g., irritable bowel syndrome; these are the most difficult to treat and are a source of frustration to patient and physician.

ANATOMY OF PAIN

Pain is produced by unpleasant *noxious* stimuli, including heat, extreme cold and mechanical injury, usually of strong intensity. At weaker intensities, these stimuli may produce other somatic sensations, i.e., warmth, cold and pressure. The perception of pain depends on the transmission of electrical impulses from the site of tissue injury in the periphery to higher centers in the brain; this is termed *nociception*. Those parts of the nervous system essential for pain transmission or nociception include: (1) pain receptors, (2) primary afferent neuronal fibers, (3) the spinothalamic tract and collateral fibers and (4) higher brain centers (Fig. 1).

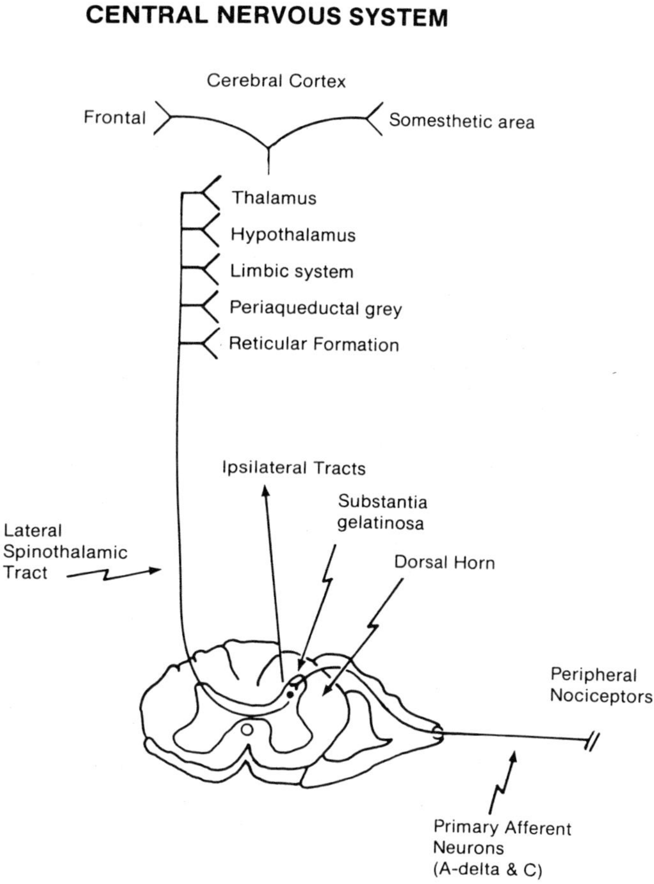

FIGURE 1. SCHEMATIC REPRESENTATION OF ANATOMICAL CONNECTIONS ASSOCIATED WITH PAIN PERCEPTION.

Receptors. Receptors that respond to noxious stimuli, thus producing electrical potentials in neurons which carry pain information to the central nervous system are termed **nociceptors**; they are free unencapsulated nerve endings. The distribution of nociceptors varies throughout the body. Areas of high nociceptor concentration include subcutaneous tissue, periosteum, deep fascia, ligaments, joint capsules and the cornea of the eye; few nociceptors are found in skeletal muscle and hardly any in bone and cartilage.

Primary Afferent Neurons. Electrical impulses are transported from nociceptors into the central nervous system via primary afferent neuronal fibers. Neurons are classified into three groups based on their cross-sectional area and speed of conduction: A fibers are the largest and the most rapid conducting, C fibers are the smallest and the slowest conducting, and B fibers are intermediate in cross-sectional area and speed of conduction. Pain is transmitted along relatively small cross-sectional neurons comprised of A-delta and C fibers. The A-delta fibers are the smallest of the A fibers, surrounded only by a thin myelin sheath and transmitting at a rate of 6 to 30 m/s. They are distributed primarily to the skin and mucous membranes. About 10 to 25% of A-delta fibers carry noxious stimuli. They respond to strong stimuli, producing a fast, sharp, easily localized pain, e.g., the pain of a finger stick with a lancet. About 50 to 70% of C fibers also transmit pain impulses; these neurons are unmyelinated and therefore conduct more slowly (0.5 to 2 m/s) and are responsible for duller, more prolonged pain. This longer lasting pain is associated with somatic and autonomic reflexes, usually sympathetic in nature (i.e., cardiac acceleration, peripheral vasoconstriction, pupillary dilatation and sweating). Nociceptors on C fibers are polymodal since they are capable of being activated by mechanical and thermal stimuli and chemical mediators of inflammation. Some receptors on A-delta fibers in skin have now been identified which act similar to the polymodal receptors normally associated with C fibers.

The peripheral afferent neurons enter the spinal cord at various levels via the dorsal roots and form cell bodies in the dorsal root ganglia. The nerves bifurcate, may ascend or descend 1 to 2 segments of the cord and give off many collaterals which are at least partially responsible for the autonomic and somatic reflexes. The primary afferent fibers terminate in the marginal layer (Lamina I), substantia gelatinosa (Lamina II and III), Lamina V and, to a smaller extent, in Lamina IV. At this point, the message is transmitted to secondary neurons, most of which cross the midline and enter the lateral spinothalamic tract. Some ipsilateral tracts also exist. The dorsal horn acts as the site by which descending pathways modulate pain.

Spinothalamic Tract Neurons. As neurons of the spinothalamic tract transverse the spinal cord, fibers are added at each segment. Spinothalamic neurons can be subdivided into (1) the neospinothalamic tract, which terminates in the ventrolateral and posterior thalamus and may be responsible for sharp, well-localized pain, and (2) the paleospinothalamic tract, which terminates in the medial thalamus and forms synapses with other neurons connecting to the reticular formation, midbrain, periaqueductal grey, limbic system and hypothalamus. These connections may help regulate respiration, endocrine function and the cardiovascular system as well as modulate descending inhibitory neurons.

Higher Brain Centers. The thalamus is the lowest level of the brain at which pain reaches consciousness; however, particularly in chronic pain, there appears to be poor localization. Pain information is disseminated from the thalamus to both cerebral hemispheres. Fibers terminate in the post-central gyrus (somesthetic area) of the parietal lobe which appears to be involved in pain discrimination, i.e., localization and intensity. Other fibers terminate in the frontal lobe which stimulates afferent fibers to the limbic system. This pathway appears to regulate the emotional or unpleasant aspect of pain. The response of the limbic system may determine how an individual responds to a noxious stimulus, adding the behavioral or subjective nature of pain. This may explain why different individuals respond differently to the same stimulus or why a single individual responds differently at various times.

Theory of Pain Perception. A very popular hypothesis to explain the perception of pain was developed by Melzack and Wall in 1965; this is commonly referred to as the Gate Theory (Fig. 2). These authors proposed that the substantia gelatinosa of the dorsal horn is an important area at which pain perception could be modulated. A "target" cell is located in the dorsal gray horn, which is stimulated by both large mechanofibers and smaller pain-conducting fibers. The "target" cell relays information to higher brain centers for pain perception. The substantia gelatinosa inhibits input from these fibers to the "target" cell. Small pain fibers inhibit the substantia gelatinosa reducing its inhibitory effect on fibers that stimulate the "target" cell; thus, pain persists. The large fibers stimulate the substantia gelatinosa, enhancing its inhibitory effect; this tends to be self-limiting and would reduce painful stimuli from the same area. This pathway may explain the "counter-irritation" theory: that by applying pressure or rubbing an area at the site of an injury, pain perception is reduced by stimulation of large mechanofibers. Higher centers also send descending inhibitory neurons which may reduce pain perception at this level of the brain. The modulatory effect of descending neurons may explain the temporary reduction in pain perception often seen in certain situations, e.g., an injured soldier performing a heroic act in a battle.

Although some of the original proposals by Melzack and Wall are highly controversial, the concept remains immensely important in any discussion of pain pathways. For example, it has been demonstrated that electrical stimulation of large afferent fibers can inhibit small primary afferent fibers. This probably explains the therapeutic effectiveness of electrical stimulation in reducing pain.

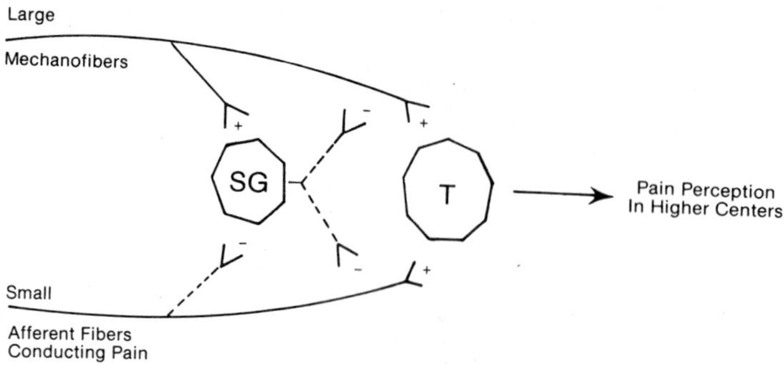

FIGURE 2. THE GATE THEORY OF PAIN PERCEPTION. *The gate theory was proposed by Melzack and Wall in 1965.* ***T*** *represents the target cell in the dorsal gray horn. Stimulation of the target cell carries impulses to higher centers for the perception of pain. The substantia gelatinosa (**SG**) inhibits fibers which would stimulate the target cell. Small afferent fibers (pain conduction) inhibit the **SG**, thus enhancing pain perception. Large sensory fibers (mechanofibers) stimulate the **SG**, thus reducing the perception of pain.*

BIOCHEMICAL MEDIATORS OF PAIN

Nociceptors are not thought to be directly stimulated by noxious stimuli. When a noxious stimulus produces tissue injury, chemical mediators are released and activate nociceptors which, in turn, generate nerve impulses. Several substances have been identified which can produce pain following intradermal administration; these include acetylcholine, histamine, potassium chloride, and polypeptides such as bradykinin and substance P. These and other substances are known to be released by a painful stimulus and may act at different levels of the pain pathway as either neurotransmitters or neuromodulators. Acetylcholine, amino acids such as aspartate and glutamate, and some peptides are involved in higher brain centers. Gamma-aminobutyric acid (GABA) and serotonin may have an important role in the spinal regulation of pain. Kinins such as bradykinin are synthesized by a cascade triggered by activated clotting factor XII. Bradykinin, histamine, and cytokines are released in the local area of tissue injury, inducing hypersensitivity and contributing to inflammation. Peptides such as calcitonin gene-related peptide and substance P are released from the peripheral terminal of C fibers. Adenosine also appears to be released from ischemic and injured tissue, activating free nerve endings, thus enhancing the response of A-delta and C fibers.

Other substances such as prostaglandins have a direct action to stimulate pain and potentiate the action of other mediators.

Evidence has accumulated supporting an important role of substance P in the pain pathway. Substance P, an undecapeptide, is a neurotransmitter at polymodal nociceptors. The peptide has been localized in the peripheral and central nervous systems; substance P is synthesized in cell bodies in dorsal root ganglia. Stimulation of C fibers releases substance P into peripheral tissues and appears to be involved in the inflammatory response. In addition, C fibers also release substance P into the cerebrospinal fluid. Particularly high concentrations of the peptide are found in the substantia gelatinosa of the dorsal gray horn and it is involved in the relay of information from the primary afferent fiber to secondary fibers.

Prostaglandins. Prostaglandins (PGs) have been shown to be modulators of activity at polymodal nociceptors and thus have an important role as mediators in pain and the inflammatory process. The prostaglandins are a group of 20-carbon oxygenated unsaturated fatty acid derivatives which possess a variety of biological effects and are important as bioregulators in many physiological and pathological states. These ubiquitous substances are not stored free in tissues, but are synthesized as a result of trauma or perturbation of cell membranes, exert their physiologic or pathologic effects, and are rapidly biotransformed to inactive products. A scheme for the endogenous formation of prostaglandins is shown in Fig. 3.

Phospholipids containing arachidonic acid are present in all cell membranes. In response to various stimuli (such as noxious stimuli), arachidonic acid is hydrolyzed from the phospholipids by phospholipase A_2, the activity of which is enhanced by an increase in intracellular calcium. Arachidonic acid is converted by the enzyme, prostaglandin endoperoxide synthase (cyclooxygenase, COX), to the unstable cyclic endoperoxides PGG_2 and PGH_2. These cyclic endoperoxides, which may produce pain by themselves, are further biotransformed to other prostaglandins, e.g., PGE_2 and $PGF_{2\alpha}$, prostacyclin (PGI_2) or thromboxanes. It is now known that there are two COX enzymes, COX1, which is constituative, and COX2, which is not constituative, but induced by mediators of inflammation.

With respect to the pain response, prostaglandins may be formed directly by the initial pain stimulus, whether thermal, chemical, or mechanical in nature, and by the action of the peripheral pain mediators, i.e., histamine, bradykinin and substance P, on membranes of surrounding tissues. Once formed, PGE_2 and PGI_2 sensitize peripheral nociceptors and produce an enhanced pain response to stimulation by the specific pain mediators. This prostaglandin-induced *hyperalgesia* appears to be more important in the duller, more prolonged pain responses mediated via C fibers. Drugs which inhibit prostaglandin formation, e.g., aspirin, ibuprofen, etc., effectively relieve pain of this origin. All of the non-steroidal

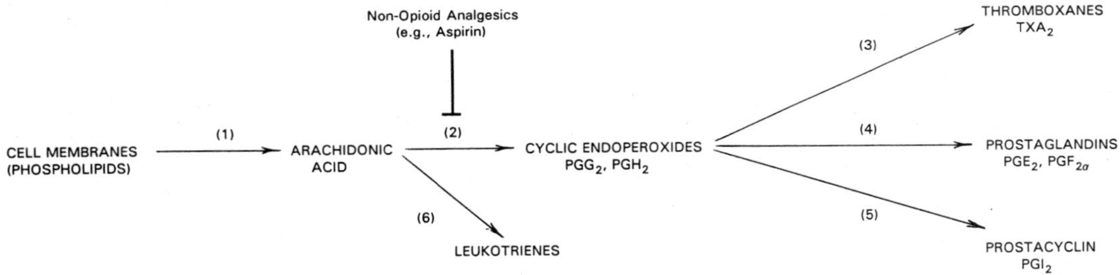

ENZYMES

(1) Phospholipase A_2
(2) Prostaglandin endoperoxide synthase (cyclooxygenase)
(3) Thromboxane synthase
(4) Isomerase and 9-keto reductase
(5) Prostacyclin synthase
(6) 5-Lipoxygenase

——┤ Inhibition

FIGURE 3. SCHEMATIC OF PROSTAGLANDIN AND LEUKOTRIENE SYNTHESIS. *The prostaglandins and leukotrienes, which are important mediators of pain and inflammation, are synthesized from phospholipids (which contain arachidonic acid) present in cell membranes. The non-opioid analgesics produce analgesia by reducing the biosynthesis and release of prostaglandins by inhibition of prostaglandin endoperoxide synthase (fatty acid cyclooxygenase).*

anti-inflammatory drugs (NSAIDs) inhibit both COX1 and COX2.

The pain associated with primary dysmenorrhea is an interesting example. Locally released PGE_2 and $PGF_{2\alpha}$ elicit strong contractions of the uterine smooth muscle; $PGF_{2\alpha}$ also causes vasoconstriction of arterioles in the tissue, leading to reduced blood flow and tissue ischemia. Thus the pain of dysmenorrhea involves (a) PGE_2- and PGI_2-induced hyperalgesia of uterine nociceptors, (b) intense muscular contractions, and (c) tissue ischemia.

Leukotrienes. Another series of compounds, the leukotrienes have also been studied and their role in the inflammatory process has been evaluated. The leukotrienes are also derivatives of arachidonic acid originally found in leukocytes (Fig. 3). They are produced by the reactions of oxygen with arachidonic acid and other polyunsaturated fatty acids, catalyzed by 5-lipoxygenase. Like the prostaglandins, leukotrienes are not stored in tissue, but upon the appropriate stimuli are rapidly synthesized and released from leukocytes and biotransformed to inactive products. These agents are important mediators of inflammation and allergic reactions by a synergistic action with other mediators such as histamine. For example, leukotriene B_4 (LTB_4) is chemotactic for leukocytes, whereas LTC_4 and LTD_4 increase vascular permeability. In the lung, LTC_4, LTD_4, and LTE_4 (components of slow-reacting substance of anaphylaxis, SRS-A) produce bronchoconstriction, and may induce asthma.

ENDOGENOUS ANALGESIC MECHANISMS

The brain contains a very important system for the regulation of pain. This was demonstrated by two findings: (1) electrical stimulation of discretely distributed loci in the brain elicits analgesia which lasts for several hours following termination of the stimulus, and (2) endogenous opioid-like substances have been identified which modulate synaptic transmission in specific areas of the brain. Today it is known that there are at least three groups of endogenous opioid peptides: enkephalins, dynorphins and β-endorphin. Each of these has its own precursor and a distinct anatomical distribution.

In addition, since 1973, three classes of opioid receptors have been identified, with specific subtypes recently cloned. The opioid receptors have been named *mu* (μ) which mediates most actions of morphine-like drugs (analgesia, respiratory depression, inhibition of gastrointestinal motility, and physical dependence); *kappa* (κ) which mediates sedation, analgesia, dysphoria, and diuresis; and *delta* (δ) which has a role in analgesia and gastrointestinal motility.

Enkephalins and Dynorphins. The enkephalins are a pair of pentapeptides, identical in structure except for the C-terminal amino acid, methionine in one (Met-enkephalin) and leucine in the other (Leu-enkephalin). Their precursor, proenkephalin, has been located in the brain, the spinal cord, and the adrenal medulla. The enkephalins are localized in areas related to pain modulation: periaqueductal grey of the midbrain, raphe magnus, substantia gelatinosa and marginal layer.

There is good correlation between opioid receptors and neurons containing enkephalin. Enkephalin-containing neurons are also highly associated with substance P-containing neurons. Enkephalins have been located in synaptosomal fractions and are rapidly inactivated by peptidases; therefore, they appear to act as neurotransmitters (Fig. 4). The proposed mechanism of enkephalin-induced analgesia is as follows: enkephalins inhibit transmission of nociception principally at the spinal cord. They are contained in short interneurons and upon release, they bind to stereospecific opioid receptors to modulate synaptic transmission; they appear to have mostly delta, with some mu, receptor activity. In the dorsal horn, they bind presynaptically to substance P-containing primary afferent fibers, reducing calcium transport across the membrane and inhibiting the release of substance P. Enkephalins may also directly alter projection neurons of the spinothalamic tract. Their role in higher centers is more complicated. Endogenous opioid peptide neurons enhance the activity of descending inhibitory neurons to the spinal cord from the periaqueductal grey and rostral medulla, presumably by inhibition of inhibitory interneurons in higher centers. Inputs to these enkephalin-containing neurons may come from ascending substance P-containing neurons or from β-endorphin-containing neurons from the pituitary or the hypothalamus.

The exact role of dynorphins in regulation of pain is less well known. Dynorphins and related substances are formed by the cleavage of a large polypeptide precursor, prodynorphin. Dynorphin A contains 17 amino acids and dynorphin B, 12 amino acids; the first five amino acids of each are identical to leu-enkephalin. There is a significant overlap with respect to the distribution of enkephalins and dynorphins in the brain, with some important differences: (1) although both groups of compounds are found in the periaqueductal grey, the dynorphins are located more ventrally, and (2) there are more neurons which contain enkephalin in the medulla. There also appears to be the coexistance of enkephalins and dynorphins in some dorsal horn neurons. Dynorphins have also been found in the posterior pituitary and hypothalamus. Similar to the enkephalins, dynorphin-containing neurons have a good correlation with opioid receptors in the brain; dynorphins act primarily at kappa opioid receptors. It has been proposed that the dynorphins might act by influencing projection neurons of the marginal layer of the spinal cord and thus secondarily affecting the descending inhibitory pathway.

The Endorphins. The enkephalins and dynorphins cannot account for all the opioid-like activity found in the brain. This led to the discovery of a larger group of endogenous opioid-like compounds, the endorphins. One of the most important members of the group is β-endorphin, a polypeptide of 31 amino acids, of which the first five are the same as met-enkephalin though it is not metabolized to met-

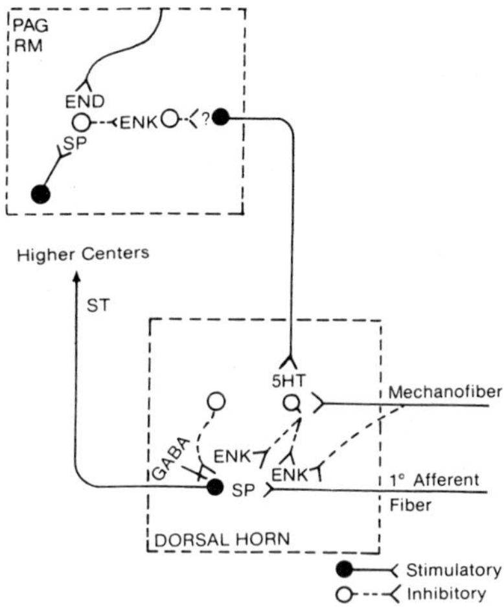

FIGURE 4. SCHEMATIC OF IMPORTANT CENTRAL NERVOUS SYSTEM PATHWAYS AND MEDIATORS OF PAIN PERCEPTION AND REGULATION. *Primary afferent neuronal fibers release substance P (**SP**) in the dorsal horn of the spinal cord, transmitting pain impulses to higher centers via the spinothalamic tract (**ST**). Release of **SP** is inhibited by enkephalin containing interneurons and directly by mechanofibers. Enkephalins (**ENK**) may also directly inhibit spinothalamic tract neurons. The activity of these **ENK** containing interneurons can be enhanced by (1) large peripheral mechanofibers, and (2) descending pathways from higher centers; a serotonergic (**5-HT**) neuron is shown as an example. Other inhibitory neurotransmitters, e.g., **GABA**, may also play an important role in pain regulation by inhibiting spinothalamic tract neurons.*

*In higher brain centers, e.g., the periaqueductal grey (**PAG**) and raphe magnus (**RM**), there are inhibitory interneurons regulating descending pathways to the dorsal horn. **ENK** containing interneurons inhibit these inhibitory interneurons, thus enhancing activity of the descending pathways. The activity of these **ENK** containing neurons is enhanced by β-endorphin (**END**) or **SP** containing neurons.*

The pathways described are a simplification; neural connections in the regulation of pain are very complex and involve the interplay of many neurons, containing and releasing a host of neurotransmitters and are not totally understood. (Modified from Basbaum and Fields, 1984).

enkephalin. β-Endorphin is synthesized in the pars intermedia and pars distalis of the pituitary and in the basal hypothalamus; it is also contained in pancreatic islet cells. This endogenous peptide is derived from pro-opiomelanocortin (POMC), a common precursor compound of adrenocorticotropic hormone (ACTH) and melanocyte-stimulating hormone. It is composed of amino acid sequence 61 to 91 of β-lipotropin. Upon painful stimuli or stress, β-endorphin is released into the bloodstream from the pituitary gland or from POMC-containing neurons which terminate in central gray matter, principally in the periaqueductal grey, where it may enhance the activity of the descending inhibitory system possibly by increasing the activity of enkephalin-containing interneurons. It has a more prolonged activity than met-enkephalin. The co-release of ACTH and β-endorphin by hypothalamic neurons may also reach the spinal cord via the cerebrospinal fluid or via POMC-containing neurons and influence spinal nociceptors directly. Pituitary endorphins may be involved in varying the threshold to pain and therefore, in pain control. In addition to analgesia, β-endorphin mimics many of the other effects of morphine including tolerance and physical dependence, respiratory depression, constipation, euphoria, and hormonal and behavioral effects and may be a mediator of the immune system. β-Endorphin acts primarily on μ and δ opioid receptors.

The anatomical circuits and biochemical mechanisms involved in pain perception and its modulation are complex and all the aspects have not been elucidated and integrated together. Figure 4 shows a schematic of some central nervous system pathways involved in pain regulation. Recent advances in pain physiology and the discovery of endogenous opioid-like compounds have provided insight toward the treatment of acute and chronic pain.

REFERENCES

Akil, H., and J.W. Lewis (Eds): *Neurotransmitters and Pain Control*, S. Karger, New York, 1987.

Drug Evaluations Annual 1993, prepared by the Department of Drugs, Division of Drugs and Toxicology, American Medical Association, Milwaukee, 1993.

Basbaum, A.I., and H.L. Fields: "Endogenous Pain Control Systems: Brainstem Spinal Pathways and Endorphin Circuitry," *Annu. Rev. Neurosci.* **7**: 309-338 (1984).

Beaumont, A., and J. Hughes: "Biology of Opioid Peptides," *Annu. Rev. Pharmacol. Toxicol.* **19**: 245-267 (1979).

Chapman, C.R., and J.J. Bonica: "Acute Pain," *Current Concepts*, Upjohn, Kalamazoo, 1983.

DiGregorio, G.J., and E.J. Barbieri: "Pharmacologic Management of Pain," *Am. Fam. Phys.* **27**: 185-188 (1983).

Fine, P.G.: "The Pathways and Mechanisms of Pain and Analgesia: A Review and Clinical Perspective," *Hosp. Formul.* **20**: 972-985 (1985).

Kelley, D.D.: "Somatic Sensory System IV: Central Representations of Pain and Analgesia," In: *Principles of Neural Science*, E.R. Kandel and J.H. Schwartz (Eds.), Elsevier North Holland, 1981, pp. 199-212.

Levine, J.: "Pain and Analgesia: The Outlook for More Rational Treatment," *Ann. Int. Med.* **100**: 269-276 (1984).

Lipman, A.G.: "Advances in Pain Management," *Hosp. Formul.* **20**: 951-985 (1985).

Loh, H.H., and A.P. Smith: "Molecular Characterization of Opioid Receptors," *Annu. Rev. Pharmacol. Toxicol.* **30**: 123-147 (1990).

Lynn, B., K. Webster, and R. Hill: "Pain," *Geigy Pharmaceuticals*, 1979.

Melzack, R., and P.D. Wall: "Pain Mechanisms: A New Theory," *Science* **150**: 971-979 (1965).

Mense, S.: "Basic Neurologic Mechanisms of Pain and Analgesia," *Am. J. Med.* **75**: 4-14 (1983).

Robinson, D.R.: "Prostaglandins, Leukotrienes and Inflammation," *Upjohn Monograph*, Kalamazoo, 1982.

Sawynok, J., and T.L. Yaksh: "Caffeine as an Analgesic Adjunct, A Review of Pharmacology and Mechanism of Action," *Pharmacol. Rev.* **45**: 43-79 (1993).

Smith, J.B.: "Prostaglandins and Related Eicosanoids," in *Basic Pharmacology in Medicine, Third Edition*, J.R. DiPalma and G.J. DiGregorio (Eds.), McGraw-Hill, New York, 1990, pp. 181-192.

Notes

PHARMACOLOGY

OF

ANALGESIC

DRUGS

METHODS OF PAIN RELIEF

Based on the current state of knowledge of the neuronal pathways and the mediators involved in the transmission of pain impulses, the perception of pain, and the endogenous analgesics peptides which are released from certain neurons to temper painful stimuli, a variety of methods have been devised to treat the patient suffering with pain. Neurological techniques and drug intervention may reduce or completely alleviate pain for many patients.

NEUROLOGICAL TECHNIQUES

The use of electrical or mechanical excitation of the nervous system by transcutaneous electrical nerve stimulation, acupuncture, neurosurgical procedures, massage, and vibration have all been used in the therapy of pain. Nerve stimulation, acupuncture and neurosurgery will be discussed briefly.

NERVE STIMULATION. Experimentally, electrical stimulation of neurons in specific areas of the central nervous system has been shown to elicit analgesia for several hours. This effect has been correlated to the release of the endogenous opioid-like substances, i.e., the endorphins, enkephalins, and dynorphins, from the appropriate neuronal tracts within the area of stimulation. Therapeutically, the use of small, battery-powered instruments such as the Transcutaneous Electrical Nerve Stimulator (TENS), placed on any part of the body, has been demonstrated to be effective in some patients with chronic pain. It appears that electrical nerve stimulation excites large mechanofibers in the periphery which, in turn, stimulate the activity of enkephalin-containing interneurons in the dorsal horn of the spinal cord resulting in analgesia.

ACUPUNCTURE. This method of analgesia, involving the insertion of fine needles into the skin and underlying muscle at various points throughout the body, was pioneered by the Chinese several thousand years ago. It has been suggested that, like electrical nerve stimulation, acupuncture needles may stimulate large afferent fibers which, upon entering the spinal cord, cause the release of endorphins and enkephalins.

NEUROSURGERY. Advances in neurosurgical methods have paralleled the progression of our understanding of pain. The neurosurgical approaches to the treatment of pain involve alteration of the activity of neuronal pathways which conduct pain impulses from the periphery to the higher brain centers. Pain relief by a neurosurgical procedure is specifically designed as a tertiary therapeutic measure; other analgesic measures should be attempted before neurosurgery is undertaken. A brief discussion of this topic is presented on pp. 73 - 76 and Tables 11 and 12.

PHARMACOTHERAPY

The use of certain types of drugs is the major method of achieving pain relief. While many drugs have analgesic properties, only certain categories of compounds can be considered useful for the relief of acute and chronic pain. For example, general anesthetics induce analgesia; however, these drugs are relatively poor analgesics except when the patient is in a semiconscious or unconscious state. The analgesia that occurs with inhalation anesthetics such as halothane (FLUOTHANE), enflurane (ETHRANE), isoflurane (FORANE), and desflurane (SUPRANE) is due to generalized central nervous system depression. In contrast, nitrous oxide is a potent analgesic at sub-anesthetic concentrations and is useful for the alleviation of pain in dental and obstetrical procedures. Therefore, with a few exceptions, these specialized drugs are not considered as important analgesics in the therapy of pain.

The use of local anesthetic agents, e.g., procaine (NOVOCAIN), lidocaine (XYLOCAINE), and bupivacaine (MARCAINE), can produce analgesia within a defined area at or near the site of injection; therefore, spinal anesthesia or peripheral nerve block can cause analgesia for short periods of time. In addition, the topical application of compounds such as benzocaine may be effective for dental pain or painful skin reactions. These drugs act by preventing the conduction and generation of nerve impulses, a process that is reversible when the drug concentration diminishes in the affected area. Although all neurons are affected by these drugs, the small diameter fibers, such as those which transmit pain (the A-delta and C fibers), are the most susceptible.

True analgesic drugs include the opioid analgesics and the non-opioid analgesics and these two categories of drugs will be discussed in detail.

ANALGESIC DRUGS

Opioid analgesics include the naturally-occurring alkaloids of opium and all of the synthetic and semi-synthetic derivatives; these drugs elicit pharmacologic effects which resemble those attributable to opium. The opioids effectively obtund severe pain through an action on the central nervous system; they also may cause euphoria, respiratory depression, sedation, constipation, emesis, miosis, and are associated with the potential to produce tolerance and physical dependence. The term *narcotic analgesics* is an older connotation for these drugs.

The *non-opioid analgesics* include the nonsteroidal anti-inflammatory drugs (NSAIDs) and the compound, acetaminophen. The NSAIDs cause a reduction in pain, fever, and inflammation. The mechanism of action associated with the analgesic, antipyretic, and anti-inflammatory effects is related to the inhibition of prostaglandin synthesis; these effects of the NSAIDs occur both peripherally and centrally. The drug, acetaminophen, has analgesic and antipyretic properties, and lacks anti-inflammatory activity. Acetaminophen is a weak inhibitor of prostaglandin synthesis.

OPIOID ANALGESICS

CLASSIFICATION. For the purposes of discussion of the pharmacologic activity of these compounds, the opioids will be classified as (1) agonists, (2) antagonists, and (3) mixed agonist-antagonists. Table 1 lists the opioid drugs which will be discussed in this and subsequent sections of the book.

MECHANISM OF ACTION. In the central nervous system there are endogenous opioid-like peptides that bind to specific receptors to produce analgesia and other effects that are similar to the opioid drugs. These endogenous substances are classified as endorphins, dynorphins, and enkephalins, and have affinity for and efficacy (the ability to stimulate the receptors and to produce an effect) at specific receptors located on cellular membranes. The receptors (designated as mu (μ), kappa (κ) and delta (δ) receptors) chemically are glycoproteins. Binding on an agonist or antagonist to these opioid receptors is stereospecific; it is the levo (-) isomer that has the higher affinity for the receptor. In addition, it has been proposed that at least two subtypes of each opioid receptor exist (e.g., mu_1 and mu_2).

Beta-endorphin binds to mu receptors, which are located primarily at supraspinal sites. The highest concentration of mu receptors is in the periaqueductal gray area. Mu receptors are associated with analgesia, euphoria, constipation, respiratory depression, and tolerance and physical dependence. Dynorphins activate kappa receptors that are found in the brain and in the spinal cord. Analgesia, miosis, tolerance, and sedation result from stimulation of these receptors. The enkephalins bind primarily to delta receptors which cause analgesia and cardiovascular effects.

Several years ago the existence of a fourth opioid receptor was postulated, i.e., the sigma (σ) receptor. The binding of certain opioids to these "receptors" (now called *sigma sites*) has been associated with dysphoria, psychotomimetic

TABLE 1. SELECTED OPIOID COMPOUNDS

CLASSIFICATION	GENERIC NAME	COMMON TRADE NAME
AGONISTS		
Phenanthrene Derivatives		
	Morphine Sulfate	
	Codeine Sulfate	
	Codeine Phosphate	
	Hydromorphone Hydrochloride	DILAUDID
	Oxymorphone Hydrochloride	NUMORPHAN
	Oxycodone Hydrochloride	
Morphinan Derivative		
	Levorphanol Tartrate	LEVO-DROMORAN
Phenylpiperidine Derivatives		
	Alfentanil Hydrochloride	ALFENTA
	Fentanyl	DURAGESIC
	Fentanyl Citrate	SUBLIMAZE
	Meperidine Hydrochloride	DEMEROL
	Sufentanil Citrate	SUFENTA
Diphenylheptane Derivatives		
	Methadone Hydrochloride	DOLOPHINE
	Propoxyphene Hydrochloride	DARVON
	Propoxyphene Napsylate	DARVON-N
ANTAGONISTS		
	Naloxone Hydrochloride	NARCAN
	Naltrexone Hydrochloride	TREXAN
MIXED AGONIST-ANTAGONISTS		
	Buprenorphine Hydrochloride	BUPRENEX
	Butorphanol Tartrate	STADOL, STADOL NS
	Dezocine	DALGAN
	Nalbuphine Hydrochloride	NUBAIN
	Pentazocine Lactate	TALWIN

effects, and respiratory stimulation. Sigma sites are not considered true opioid receptors since a number of different compounds (e.g., antipsychotics, certain antihistamines, some steroids, and phencyclidine), none of which are opioid in structure, have binding affinity for these sites.

The centrally-acting analgesic drugs (*opioid agonists*) attach to opioid receptors and mimic the activity of the endogenous opioid peptides. When pain is perceived, it appears that substance P and glutamate are the primary nociceptive transmitters that are involved in the brain and spinal cord. Substance P augments the effects of glutamate at the N-methyl-D-aspartate (NMDA) receptor and it is mainly these two neurotransmitters that modulate and cause ascending and descending pain transmission in the spinal cord and brain. Since endogenous opioid receptors are found in the same areas as is substance P, it is suggested that the analgesic action of opioid drugs is due to the fact that opioids decrease the release of substance P.

When morphine and the other opioid analgesics bind to mu, kappa, and delta receptors there occurs an increase in the influx of potassium ions into the cell which promotes hyperpolarization and a decrease of calcium ion entrance into the cell. By these actions, the opioid analgesics prevent the release of substance P and the excitatory neurotransmitter, glutamate. In addition, these drugs activate adrenergic and serotonergic neurons that inhibit the transmission of pain from the nociceptive stimulus. Other mediators such as bradykinin, somatostatin, and aspartate appear to be involved in nociceptive transmission and in some manner their effect are blocked or modified by the administration of opioid analgesic drugs.

The *opioid antagonists* bind to all three categories of opioid receptor sites throughout the body, but fail to activate them. These compounds are not used for analgesia; rather, the therapeutic use of these drugs lies in their ability to reverse the adverse effects associated with an overdose of an agonist opioid or to prevent the effects of opioids in individuals who abuse these drugs.

The compounds that comprise the *mixed agonist-antagonist group* are semi-synthetic derivatives of morphine, the chemical structures of which have (1) agonistic activity at some kappa receptors but antagonistic activity at mu receptors, e.g., pentazocine, butorphanol, and nalbuphine, or (2) partial agonistic activity at mu receptors and antagonistic activity at kappa receptors, e.g., buprenorphine. All are effective analgesics since they stimulate either mu or kappa receptors. Table 2 shows a listing of representative opioid agonists, antagonists, and mixed agonist-antagonists and the receptor(s) to which they bind.

AGONISTS. Chemically, the opioid agonists include a number of structurally different classes of drugs, all of which have pharmacologic effects similar to those of morphine. These include the phenanthrene derivatives, which encompass both

TABLE 2. OPIOID RECEPTOR BINDING OF REPRESENTATIVE OPIOID AGONISTS, ANTAGONISTS, AND AGONIST-ANTAGONISTS

DRUG	OPIOID RECEPTOR TYPES		
	Mu (μ)	Kappa (κ)	Delta (δ)
AGONISTS			
Morphine[a]	Agonist	Agonist	Agonist
ANTAGONISTS			
Naloxone	Antagonist	Antagonist	Antagonist
Naltrexone	Antagonist	Antagonist	Antagonist
MIXED AGONIST-ANTAGONISTS			
Pentazocine	Antagonist	Agonist	------[b]
Nalbuphine	Antagonist	Agonist	-------
Butorphanol	Antagonist	Agonist	-------
Buprenorphine	Partial Agonist	Antagonist	-------

[a] All of the opioids of the agonist type listed in Table 1 bind to and activate mu, kappa, and delta receptors similar to morphine. However, differences exist with respect to the degree of activity at each opioid receptor category; these drugs have greater affinity for mu than for kappa or delta receptors.

[b] ------- indicates that no significant activity has been observed or the experimental data are inadequate to define the receptor binding activity.

the naturally occurring alkaloids of opium (e.g., morphine and codeine), and their semi-synthetic derivatives (e.g., hydromorphone, oxycodone and oxymorphone), a morphinan derivative (levorphanol), phenylpiperidine derivatives (alfentanil, fentanyl, meperidine and sufentanil), and diphenylheptane derivatives (methadone and propoxyphene). Although morphine is the oldest known drug of this class, it remains as the prototype for the group and the standard to which all other opioid analgesic compounds are compared. The following discussion will review the pharmacologic effects of the opioid agonists in general with specific comparisons of the various compounds made against morphine.

Effects on Organ Systems. Although the predominant effect of the opioid agonists is the abolition of pain, these drugs have profound pharmacologic activity throughout the body. Not only is the central nervous system affected by these drugs, but peripheral systems such as the respiratory and gastrointestinal systems may show significant alterations in their normal activities.

Central Nervous System. Analgesia, drowsiness, alteration in mood and mental clouding are characteristic effects of opioids on the central nervous system. Pain relief appears to be related to drug activity at both mu and kappa receptors, and despite the fact that all of the opioid agonists stimulate these receptors, differences in potency to induce analgesia among the compounds varies greatly (see Table 3). Drowsiness occurs both in pain-free individuals and in patients experiencing pain; however, in contrast to many other types of drugs, the opioids relieve pain without a loss of consciousness. Furthermore, pain relief with the opioids is selective in that other sensations, e.g., touch, vision and hearing, are usually unaffected.

Euphoria may be experienced in 10 to 20 percent of patients, especially as pain is alleviated; however, dysphoric reactions may also occur. Lethargy, an inability to concentrate, and apathy may occur, more commonly in pain-free individuals. Opioids have excitatory and convulsant properties and should be used with caution in patients with seizure disorders.

Respiration. Morphine and the other opioid analgesics have a direct depressant effect on the brain stem respiratory centers resulting in reduced respiratory rate, minute volume and tidal exchange; irregular and periodic breathing may also occur. These effects are observable at therapeutic doses of the opioids and increase as the dose administered is raised. The respiratory depression by opioids is produced by reducing the sensitivity of the medullary chemoreceptors to carbon dioxide. Death from the overdose of an opioid is almost always the result of respiratory depression and arrest.

Nausea and Vomiting. Direct stimulation of the chemoreceptor trigger zone (CTZ) in the area postrema of the medulla causes nausea and emesis; however, a vestibular component is also involved since there is a high incidence of nausea and vomiting in ambulatory patients and this rarely occurs in bed-ridden individuals.

Pupil. Morphine and most of its derivatives constrict the pupil; this miotic effect occurs through stimulation of the autonomic portion of the nucleus of the oculomotor nerve and is a useful diagnostic sign of opioid use or abuse. Tolerance generally does not develop to opioid-induced miosis. Meperidine, however, may produce mydriasis.

Cough Reflex. Although morphine is a moderately potent depressant of the medullary-pontine cough (tussive) center, the potential for dependence and

TABLE 3. POTENCY COMPARISONS OF SELECTED OPIOID ANALGESICS[a]

DRUG	EQUIANALGESIC DOSES (mg) PO	IM	ORAL : PARENTERAL DOSE RATIO
AGONISTS			
Morphine	60	10	6.0
Codeine	200	120	1.7
Fentanyl	------[c]	0.1	------
Hydromorphone	7.5	1.5	5.0
Levorphanol	4	2	2.0
Meperidine	300	75	4.0
Methadone	20	10	2.0
Oxycodone	30	------[c]	------
Oxymorphone	10[d]	1	10.0
Propoxyphene	130	------[c]	------
Sufentanil	------[c]	0.02	------
MIXED AGONIST-ANTAGONISTS			
Buprenorphine	------[c]	0.3	------
Butorphanol	------[c]	2	------
Dezocine	------[c]	10	------
Nalbuphine	------[c]	10	------
Pentazocine	150	30	5.0

[a] The data in this Table are based upon morphine, 10 mg, administered intramuscularly and represent the general consensus of medical opinion. Variability will occur among patients; therefore, these values should be used only as a guide for comparison.

[b] These data were calculated as the ratio of the PO : IM equianalgesic doses of the compounds. The equianalgesic doses were estimated from dose-response curves and are based on the analgesic efficacy of the drugs. These data are not reflective of bioavailability which is based upon plasma concentrations of the drugs.

[c] Not used by this route.

[d] Rectal administration.

respiratory depression severely limits the antitussive benefit that may be provided by this and many other opioids. Some analgesic (e.g., codeine, hydrocodone, and hydromorphone) and non-analgesic (e.g., dextromethorphan) opioid compounds, which have high antitussive activity and a lower dependence liability, are more suitable as cough suppressants. These drugs raise the threshold for stimulation of the tussive center.

Cardiovascular System. Arteriolar vasodilatation and reduced peripheral resistance may occur with therapeutic doses of these drugs. While these effects are insignificant when patients are supine, upon standing, orthostatic hypotension and fainting may occur. Most opioid analgesics promote histamine release from mast cells and basophils, which probably participates in the hypotensive effect of these compounds. Opioids also reduce sympathetic tone to the vasculature by depression of the medullary vasomotor center. Cardiac function is not significantly affected in normal individuals; however, in patients with coronary artery disease or myocardial infarction, a decrease in oxygen consumption, left ventricular end-diastolic pressure, and cardiac work may occur.

Gastrointestinal Tract. Opioids cause constipation as a result of both peripheral and central actions. Peripherally, these compounds decrease propulsive peristaltic activity (motility) of the small intestine (the duodenum is affected more than the ileum) and the colon. Tone of the gastrointestinal sphincter muscles is usually enhanced and digestive secretions along the entire alimentary canal are reduced. The delay in the movement of bowel contents leads to desiccation of the feces which further reduces its passage through the intestine. Generalized central nervous system depression decreases perception of normal sensory stimuli arising in the rectum (defecation reflex) and enhances the local constipating effect of the drug. Also, opioids decrease the release of substance P in the myenteric plexuses which regulates intestinal peristalsis.

Although constipation constitutes an unpleasant adverse effect of most of these drugs in the therapy of pain, certain opioid derivatives [e.g., difenoxin (MOTOFEN), diphenoxylate (LOMOTIL), and loperamide (IMODIUM)] are useful for the therapy of diarrhea and are not used as analgesic agents.

Other Smooth Muscle. With the exception of vascular smooth muscle, most other smooth muscle is contracted by morphine and its congeners. Bronchiolar smooth muscle contraction can be significance; morphine can induce an asthmatic attack. Contraction of the gall bladder, bile duct and sphincter of Oddi compromise the use of morphine in pain associated with biliary colic, and contraction of vesicourethral smooth muscle may lead to urinary retention. At equianalgesic doses the effect of codeine and meperidine on the bile duct is less than that of morphine.

Skin. Therapeutic doses of the agonist opioids cause histamine release from mast cells and basophils, which is partially responsible for the cutaneous vasodilation, pruritic, and sweating that may occur following the administration of these drugs. Opioid-induced histamine release is a chemical interaction whereby the drug displaces histamine from binding sites in mast cells. It resembles, and may be confused with, allergic reactions.

Tolerance and Physical Dependence. Both of these conditions impose major limitations to the continued use of opioid agonists for chronic pain. Tolerance occurs when the same dose of a drug elicits a decreased effect following repeated administration, or when increasingly greater doses are required to achieve the effect observed with the initial dose of the drug. Physical dependence is a condition produced by continued dosing with a drug, in which an alteration in the physiological state of the individual results and the continued use of the compound (or a structurally-related derivative) is needed in order to prevent the appearance of withdrawal reactions.

Tolerance does not occur equally to all of the effects of the opioids. Most commonly, patients become tolerant to the effects mediated predominantly via the central nervous system, i.e., analgesia, euphoria and dysphoria, sedation, respiratory depression, nausea and vomiting, and cough suppression. However, tolerance is minimal or does not occur at all to the constipating effect or pupillary effects of these drugs. In addition, it is important to realize that the rapidity with which tolerance occurs is both dose and time dependent. Large amounts of a drug with short intervals between doses induce tolerance faster than small doses administered farther apart. In general, tolerance to the opioid analgesics does not become clinically-relevant until 2 to 3 weeks of continual administration of therapeutic doses.

As a group, the opioid agonists have a high potential for the production of physical dependence following chronic use. Similar to tolerance, the time required to produce physical dependence following chronic administration varies considerably and is somewhat related to the amount of drug administered, but may be as short as 1 to 2 weeks if large quantities of drug are used. Cross-dependence, i.e., within the opioid group, is common. Table 4 lists many of the signs and symptoms of withdrawal to morphine and the other agonist opioid analgesics. There is evidence to support the belief that the abuse liability of the agonist-antagonist opioids is less than with the agonist compounds; this will be discussed later in the text.

Pharmacokinetics. The agonist opioids are readily absorbed from the gastrointestinal tract following oral administration and also after either subcutaneous or intramuscular injection; rectal administration results in adequate absorption and a few compounds (i.e., morphine, hydromorphone and oxymorphone) are available in rectal suppositories. Fentanyl is available in a transdermal system which is applied to the skin and provides pain relief for 72

TABLE 4. SIGNS AND SYMPTOMS OF OPIOID WITHDRAWAL[a]

HOURS AFTER LAST DOSE	SIGNS AND SYMPTOMS[b,c]	
8 to 12	Lacrimation Rhinorrhea	Yawning Sweating
12 to 14	Restless ("Yen") Sleep	
18 to 20	Dilated Pupils Anorexia Gooseflesh Tremors	Restlessness Irritability Anxiety
48 to 72 (Peak)	Increased Irritability Insomnia Marked Anorexia Violent Yawning Severe Sneezing Lacrimation Coryza Muscle Spasms Generalized Body Aches	Nausea and Vomiting Diarrhea Abdominal Cramping Increased Heart Rate Increased Blood Pressure Chills and Hyperthermia Flushing Low Back Pain Hyperpnea

Duration of the withdrawal syndrome is approximately 7 to 10 days.

[a] For morphine and other mu receptor agonists with durations of action similar to morphine.

[b] The signs and symptoms of meperidine withdrawal usually begin to appear within 3 hours after the last dose, peak in 8 to 12 hours, and then decline; the duration is approximately 4 to 5 days. Lacrimation, rhinorrhea, sweating, pupillary dilation, nausea, vomiting and diarrhea are generally less severe than morphine; however, muscle spasms, restlessness, anxiety and irritability may be more intense.

[c] The methadone abstinence syndrome presents signs and symptoms similar to those listed above; however, the condition develops more slowly (24 to 48 hours after the last dose), is more prolonged (peak of 1 to 3 weeks; duration up to 6 to 7 weeks), and is usually less intense than the morphine withdrawal.

hours with a single application. The oral bioavailability of most of these opioids is less than 60 percent, since hepatic first-pass biotransformation will reduce the amount of compound that will be made available to the entire body. Morphine, for example, has an average oral bioavailability of approximately 15 to 20 percent; however, this may range from 10 to 50 percent, indicating that considerable variability does exist among patients. In general, the effective oral dose is greater than the parenteral dose, resulting in a high oral : parenteral dose ratio (see Table 3); however, this is also quite variable among patients and also depends on the particular compound. Codeine, levorphanol, and methadone have a lower first-pass biotransformation and a lower oral : parenteral dose ratio.

Most of the opioids are biotransformed to inactive glucuronide conjugates in the liver; however, a few active biotransformation products can be formed. For example, morphine-6-glucuronide is a potent analgesic; normeperidine is about half as active as an analgesic as its parent meperidine; and approximately 10 percent of codeine, the 3-methyl derivative of morphine, is demethylated to morphine prior to inactivation. Over 90 percent of an administered dose of an opioid is excreted in the urine as inactive metabolites; the remainder appears in the feces via biliary excretion, mainly as the more lipid-soluble parent drug. Enterohepatic recirculation of the active moiety will occur with all of these drugs to a small extent. Metabolites of morphine are also detected in saliva.

Following intramuscular injection, the agonist opioids have an onset of the analgesic effect within 30 minutes and a peak effect within 90 minutes. The plasma half-life of these drugs is generally within 4 hours, although methadone (due to high plasma protein binding) has a plasma half-life of approximately 1 day, levorphanol (due to slower metabolism) has a plasma half-life of about 11 hours, and propoxyphene (due to highly variable, but generally slow systemic clearance) has a half-life between 6 and 12 hours. Table 5 summarizes some of the pharmacokinetic information available concerning these drugs.

ANTAGONISTS. Naloxone and naltrexone are competitive antagonists of both the agonist opioids and the mixed agonist-antagonist compounds at all opioid receptor sites; therefore, they effectively prevent or reverse all of the pharmacologic effects produced by these drugs. Both naloxone and naltrexone are "pure" antagonists, i.e., they lack agonistic activity at opioid receptors. Neither of these compounds produce analgesia, respiratory depression, pupillary constriction or psychotomimetic effects. Furthermore, neither tolerance nor physical dependence have been observed with these drugs.

Pharmacokinetics. Naloxone is a relatively short-acting drug; the plasma half-life is approximately 1 hour in adults and 3 hours in neonates. Although the compound is absorbed following oral administration, first-pass biotransformation by hepatic glucuronide conjugation is so rapid that tissue concentrations are

TABLE 5. SOME PHARMACOKINETIC DATA OF OPIOID ANALGESICS

DRUG	ONSET OF EFFECT[a] (MINUTES)	PEAK EFFECT[a] (MINUTES)	DURATION OF EFFECT (HOURS)	PLASMA HALF-LIFE (HOURS)
AGONISTS				
Morphine	30	30 to 90	3 to 7	2 to 3
Alfentanil	------[b]	------------[b]	0.5 to 1	1 to 2
Codeine	30	45 to 90	4 to 6	3 to 4
Fentanyl	10	20 to 30	1 to 2	3 to 4
Hydromorphone	30	30 to 90	4 to 5	2 to 4
Levorphanol	30	60 to 90	4 to 8	10 to 12
Meperidine	15	30 to 60	2 to 4	3 to 4
Methadone	15	60 to 120	4 to 6	21 to 25
Oxycodone[c]	15	45 to 60	4 to 6	-----------[b]
Oxymorphone	10	30 to 90	3 to 6	-----------[b]
Propoxyphene[c]	60	60 to 90	4 to 6	6 to 12
Sufentanil	5	------------[b]	------------[b]	2 to 3
MIXED AGONIST-ANTAGONISTS				
Buprenorphine	15	45 to 60	4 to 6	2 to 3
Butorphanol	10	30 to 60	3 to 4	2 to 4
Dezocine	30	30 to 150	2 to 4	---------[b]
Nalbuphine	15	45 to 60	3 to 6	4 to 6
Pentazocine	15	30 to 60	2 to 3	2 to 3

[a] Based on intramuscular administration.

[b] No data available.

[c] Based on oral administration.

inadequate to produce the desired effect; therefore, the drug must be used parenterally. The onset of action is generally within 2 minutes following an IV dose; IM administration results in a slightly longer onset time. The drug and its inactive metabolites are excreted in the urine. Due to the rapid inactivation of the compound (the mean plasma half-life is approximately 1 hour in adults), the duration of action is limited to 1 to 4 hours after IV use and 2 to 5 hours after SC or IM administration. Slower hepatic glucuronidation by neonates results in a longer plasma half-life (approximately 3 hours) and a longer duration of action.

Naltrexone is an opioid receptor antagonist that offers the advantages of oral activity and a long duration of action, i.e., 24 to 72 hours. Like naloxone, this drug undergoes extensive first-pass biotransformation; however, the major metabolite, 6-β-naltrexol, is also a pure competitive opioid antagonist like the parent compound but weaker in its effect. Although naltrexone has a mean plasma half-life of 4 hours and does not accumulate during chronic administration, 6-β-naltrexol (plasma half-life = 13 hours) will accumulate in the body after continued use and is, in part, responsible for the long duration of action observed with naltrexone. Both compounds are excreted primarily via the urine.

Therapeutic Uses. Since these compounds lack significant analgesic activity, they are not used for the therapy of pain. Naloxone is indicated for the complete or partial reversal of opioid-induced depression including respiratory depression in emergency room settings and has also been used for the diagnosis of suspected opioid intoxication. In contrast, naltrexone is indicated as an adjunct to the maintenance of detoxified, formerly opioid-dependent subjects in an opioid-free state. Naloxone will block the effects of heroin or other opioids that the individual tries to abuse.

MIXED AGONIST-ANTAGONISTS. The mixed agonist-antagonist opioids include buprenorphine, butorphanol, dezocine, nalbuphine, and pentazocine and all of these compounds possess properties of both the aforementioned groups of opioids. They differ from the pure opioid agonists and antagonists in that they show opioid receptor selectivity, i.e., they may stimulate one type of opioid receptor while blocking another (see Table 2). All five of these drugs are potent, effective analgesics (through an agonistic action at either mu or kappa receptors) and they may induce adverse effects typically associated with the opioid agonists, i.e., respiratory depression, nausea and vomiting, and constipation. Their advantages lie in (1) less respiratory depression at therapeutic analgesic doses and (2) a lower dependence liability as compared to the opioid agonist group.

Similar to naloxone and naltrexone, these drugs may demonstrate their antagonistic activity at opioid receptors in individuals with opioid dependence by precipitating withdrawal symptoms. Buprenorphine is a potent opioid antagonist that is approximately equipotent with naloxone; however, the other drugs are weak antagonists; for example, butorphanol, nalbuphine, and pentazocine are only 1/40, 1/100, and 1/1000 as potent as opioid receptor antagonists in comparison to naloxone and, therefore, should not be used for this purpose.

Pharmacokinetics. Representative pharmacokinetic data for these compounds are summarized in Table 5. Similar to the other opioids, these drugs are biotransformed in the liver and excreted in the urine.

DRUG MONOGRAPHS. The following drug monographs contain additional information concerning each of the opioid analgesics mentioned above. Following the monograph on morphine sulfate, the prototype of the opioid analgesics, monographs on the other opioid analgesics are arranged alphabetically by the generic name of the drug. The pharmaceutical preparations that are available, common adult and pediatric dosages, and routes of administration are listed in Table D (pp. 114 - 119) and Table K (pp. 140 - 143).

Morphine Sulfate. Morphine is usually employed parenterally for the rapid, effective relief of pain. Oral preparations of morphine sulfate are available, but are less potent than the injectable forms since only 15 to 20 percent of an oral dose reaches the systemic circulation. There are controlled (sustained) release tablets of morphine sulfate, e.g., MS CONTIN, ROXANOL SR, which release the drug from the tablet more slowly than from the conventional (immediate release) oral morphine preparations. The oral bioavailability of the drug using these controlled release dosage forms is approximately 40 percent; however, the rate of absorption is slower with these products. Morphine sulfate is well-distributed throughout the body (the apparent volume of distribution is approximately 3.3 L/kg) but only small amounts pass the blood-brain barrier in contrast to the more lipid soluble compounds, e.g., codeine and methadone. The liver is the site of biotransformation of this compound to an active metabolite, morphine-6-glucuronide, and the inactive product, morphine-3-glucuronide.

Therapeutic plasma concentrations of morphine have been estimated between 75 and 150 ng/mL; elderly patients may have higher plasma drug concentrations and may show a greater susceptibility to adverse effects of the drug. When morphine sulfate is given using either the immediate release preparations or the controlled release tablets on a fixed dosing regimen, a steady state plasma concentration is achieved in about 24 hours. For any fixed dose and dosing interval the controlled release tablets will provide, at the steady state, a lower maximum average plasma concentration and a higher minimum average plasma concentration than the conventional oral morphine. This is a potential advantage by reducing fluctuations in plasma levels over dosing intervals. The activity of opium is primarily due to the morphine content of the substance and pharmaceutical preparations containing opium, e.g., paregoric (camphorated tincture of opium), are available for use as analgesics or antidiarrheals.

Alfentanil Hydrochloride (ALFENTA). This compound, a derivative of fentanyl, is used as an IV analgesic adjunct given in incremental doses or by continuous infusion in the maintenance of general anesthesia in combination with nitrous oxide/oxygen or barbiturate/nitrous oxide/oxygen. The drug can also be used as a primary anesthetic for the induction of anesthesia when endotracheal intubation and assisted ventilation are necessary. Blood concentrations of 100 to 200 ng/mL are effective for superficial surgery, while 300 to 350 ng/mL are reported necessary to induce anesthesia for abdominal surgery. The pharmacologic effects of alfentanil hydrochloride are similar to morphine sulfate, except that there appears to be less respiratory depression and little evidence of histamine release. Similar to its congener fentanyl, rapid IV injection will induce an increase in skeletal muscle tone. Alfentanil is about 1/10th the potency of fentanyl. The pharmacokinetics of the drug can be very variable among patients; typically the elimination half-life of the drug ranges from 1 to 2 hours following IV use. Over 99 percent of an administered dose is biotransformed in the liver and eliminated via the urine.

Buprenorphine Hydrochloride (BUPRENEX). This drug is a mixed agonist-antagonist opioid that induces pharmacologic effects qualitatively similar to those of morphine sulfate. It is used for moderate to severe pain. Interestingly, the drug appears to be a partial agonist at mu receptors, i.e., it has both agonistic and antagonistic activity depending upon the dose, and it dissociates from these receptors very slowly. Consequently, once the effects of this drug have been produced, they are not easily reversed by opioid antagonists like naloxone. Decreased respiratory rate and depth has been claimed to be less severe than equianalgesic doses of morphine; however, there have been reports of clinically significant respiratory depression with this drug. In doses higher than recommended for pain relief, the drug shows increased antagonistic activity; therefore, the use of buprenorphine in opioid-dependent individuals may lead to symptoms of withdrawal. While this compound has been used parenterally, orally, and sublingually, it is only available for use by injection in the United States at the present time.

Butorphanol Tartrate (STADOL). Butorphanol is a potent opioid analgesic that acts primarily at kappa receptors; some experimental data suggest that the drug has weak antagonistic activity at mu receptors. This opioid is used intravenously or intramuscularly for analgesia. A nasal spray preparation (STADOL NS) is available for the treatment of pain associated with migraine headaches. Respiratory depression is observed at high therapeutic doses of butorphanol tartrate, but a ceiling effect occurs rapidly in the degree of respiratory depression produced. Studies have shown that this agent has a low dependence liability and, in contrast to most other opioid analgesics, it is not classified under the Controlled Substances Act (for a brief discussion of this Act and a listing of drugs contained in its regulatory schedules, see pp. 107 - 108).

Codeine Sulfate and Codeine Phosphate. Codeine is usually administered orally either alone or in combination with non-opioid analgesics such as aspirin or acetaminophen for mild to moderate pain. It is also an effective antitussive agent. Codeine has more of a stimulant effect on the central nervous system than morphine. This stimulatory effect of codeine is due to the formation of the metabolite norcodeine. Codeine salts are well-absorbed orally and have a higher oral bioavailability than morphine; this is reflected by the fact that codeine has the lowest oral : parenteral dose ratio of all the opioid analgesics (see Table 3). When used by injection, codeine has few advantages over morphine as an analgesic. The liability for drug dependence with this compound appears to be less than that of morphine; however, at equianalgesic doses, codeine induces greater histamine release than morphine, leading to a greater incidence of hypotension, cutaneous vasodilation, urticaria, and bronchoconstriction.

Dihydrocodeine bitartrate is a derivative of codeine that is also available for use as an analgesic. This drug has the same pharmacologic properties as codeine. Presently dihydrocodeine is only available for oral administration and is marketed in a fixed combination with aspirin and caffeine (as SYNALGOS-DC).

Dezocine (DALGAN). This drug is a synthetic opioid agonist-antagonist and appears to have greater affinity for mu receptors than kappa receptors. The analgesic potency and the pharmacokinetics of dezocine are comparable to morphine sulfate. The drug is used only by the IM and IV routes. Effective analgesia in patients with postoperative pain occurs at serum concentrations above 5 to 9 ng/mL. Most of the compound is biotransformed by glucuronide conjugation and these inactive metabolites are excreted in the urine. In patients with kidney or liver impairment the dosage of dezocine should be decreased. The pharmacologic effects of dezocine are similar to other agonist-antagonist opioids and although respiratory depression has been observed, a ceiling effect occurs rapidly in the degree of respiratory depression produced. Like butorphanol tartrate, dezocine appears to have a very low potential for abuse; consequently it is not regulated under the Controlled Substances Act.

Fentanyl Citrate (SUBLIMAZE). Although this compound is structurally related to meperidine hydrochloride, a drug that is a potent mu receptor and kappa receptor stimulant, fentanyl is primarily a mu receptor agonist and one of the most potent opioid analgesics. The respiratory depressant effect of the drug is of shorter duration than meperidine and the emetic activity is less than with equianalgesic doses of either morphine or meperidine. Little histamine release occurs in doses up to 50 μg/kg. Rapid IV injection or high IM doses will induce an increase in skeletal muscle tone believed to be mediated through an alteration in dopaminergic activity in the striatum. Fentanyl citrate alone is indicated for use as an analgesic during anesthesia. Following IV administration, the onset of action is immediate and the duration is usually between 30 and 60 minutes; after IM use the onset of action is 7 to 8 minutes and the effects last 1 to 2 hours. The effective plasma concentration of fentanyl citrate is about 1 ng/mL for postoperative analgesia, but 3 ng/mL appears to be required for effective intraoperative analgesia. This drug is often combined with a neuroleptic such as droperidol for neuroleptanalgesia and with droperidol and nitrous oxide for neuroleptanesthesia.

Fentanyl Transdermal System (DURAGESIC). This dosage form of fentanyl provides for continuous delivery of drug for 72 hours. When the transdermal system is applied to the skin, fentanyl moves from the reservoir across the copolymer release membrane through the skin and into the circulation. The peak concentration of fentanyl in the serum is reached between 24 and 72 hours after application. Following removal of the device from the skin, it takes between 13 and 22 hours for the serum level of fentanyl to decline to 50 percent of its value when the transdermal system was removed. There are 4 systems available that contain 2.5, 5.0, 7.5, and 10.0 mg and provide for a rate of delivery of 25, 50, 75, and 100 μg/hr, respectively. The required dosage should be individually determined for each patient. Caution should be used if the transdermal system is applied to a number of patients such as those with bradycardia, liver impairment, renal dysfunction fever, and those patients who are elderly or debilitated. Fentanyl is a potent opioid analgesic. The fentanyl transdermal system is indicated in the management of chronic pain. Careful titration of the dose can reduce or prevent the occurrence of adverse reactions generally seen with opioid agonists.

Hydrocodone Bitartrate (HYCODAN). This is a semisynthetic opioid analgesic and antitussive with pharmacologic activity similar to that of codeine. When used alone it is generally indicated for the relief of cough, rarely for the relief of pain. For its analgesic effects it is more commonly combined with aspirin or acetaminophen.

Hydromorphone Hydrochloride (DILAUDID). The effects of this morphine derivative are qualitatively identical to morphine sulfate; the drug is approximately 8 times more potent than morphine on a milligram basis, however. It is used to treat moderate to severe pain. Although commonly used orally and by SC or IM injection, hydromorphone hydrochloride can be used by slow IV administration. Rectal suppositories are also available and may be useful in some patients. Since this compound is more water-soluble than morphine sulfate and higher concentrations may be injected in small volumes, hydromorphone is quite useful in emaciated patients requiring large IM doses. In addition, the drug is a very effective antitussive agent and is available for oral administration for this purpose; however, the high dependence liability of the compound makes it less useful as an antitussive than other drugs.

Levomethadyl Acetate Hydrochloride (ORLAAM). This opioid agonist is indicated for the treatment of opioid addiction similar to the use of methadone in the management of opioid dependence. This compound is not to be used outside of an approved drug treatment program. Levomethadyl acetate is available as a 10 mg/mL solution. After determining the dosage, the drug is diluted with liquid prior to oral administration. There are suggested doses for initial treatment and for maintenance dosage. The drug is given 3 times a week. Every-other-day dosing, however, may be necessary in some cases. Caution should be exercised when determining the required dosage to prevent overdosage. Levomethadyl acetate has the same pharmacological effects as do other opioid agonists such as sedation, respiratory depression, and reduction of cardiovascular function.

Levorphanol Tartrate (LEVO-DROMORAN). The pharmacological effects of this drug are similar to morphine sulfate except that the incidence of nausea, vomiting and constipation are reported to be less than with the prototype agent. By IM injection levorphanol tartrate is approximately 5 times more potent than morphine sulfate and, like codeine, has a low oral : parenteral dose ratio. The onset and peak analgesic effects are comparable to morphine; however, the duration of the analgesia is somewhat longer since levorphanol is biotransformed less rapidly, resulting is a longer elimination half-life (see Table 5).

Meperidine Hydrochloride (DEMEROL). Meperidine is a highly effective and commonly used synthetic analgesic that binds strongly to both mu receptors and kappa receptors. As noted previously, it is less potent than morphine (see Table 3). Most of the pharmacologic effects of this drug are similar to morphine sulfate with the following exceptions: (1) meperidine (in high doses) may cause central nervous system excitation, characterized by tremors, multifocal myoclonus, and seizures, (2) it induces a lower incidence of constipation than morphine, (3) it has antimuscarinic activity, and (4) the drug has little effect on the cough reflex. Meperidine hydrochloride is adequately absorbed following oral administration (the bioavailability is about 50 percent) and distributed similar to most opioids (the volume of distribution is about 4.4 L/kg). Effective plasma concentrations range between 100 and 800 ng/mL with a mean of between 400 and 500 ng/mL. Meperidine appears to be slightly more rapidly acting than morphine and its biotransformation is more complex. One of its metabolites, normeperidine, is about one-half as active as an analgesic as the parent compound and the excitatory symptoms observed following large doses of meperidine appears to be due to the accumulation of this biotransformation product. The half-life of normeperidine has been estimated to be between 15 and 20 hours; therefore, compromised renal or hepatic function increases the possibility of the appearance of the central nervous system stimulatory effects.

Methadone Hydrochloride (DOLOPHINE). Although this synthetic compound differs chemically from morphine sulfate, it is an effective mu receptor agonist with pharmacologic effects similar to those of morphine sulfate. Methadone hydrochloride is effective both parenterally and orally and has an oral bioavailability of over 90 percent. It is highly bound to plasma and tissue proteins (about 90 percent at therapeutic doses) and it is extensively biotransformed in the liver to inactive products prior to excretion in the bile and urine. The pharmacokinetics of methadone become noteworthy because the drug has a long biological half-life (up to 40 hours in some studies), will accumulate on repeated administration, and will maintain low plasma concentrations following cessation of use. Patients with reduced renal or hepatic function should be monitored carefully for signs of drug accumulation or toxicity. The long biological half-life probably accounts for the mild, but prolonged, withdrawal syndrome if drug use is stopped abruptly. Methadone is used in the treatment of severe pain. In addition, it is indicated for detoxification of, and for maintenance programs for, opioid-dependent individuals.

Nalbuphine Hydrochloride (NUBAIN). Nalbuphine is chemically related to oxymorphone and naloxone and is classified as a mixed agonist-antagonist. The drug produces analgesia by stimulation of kappa receptors and has antagonistic activity at mu receptors. Most of the pharmacologic effects of the drug are similar to morphine sulfate, except that respiratory depression attains a ceiling effect at high therapeutic doses whereas morphine does not. The respiratory depressant effect of nalbuphine is antagonized by naloxone. The half-life of this drug is 5 hours and its duration of action is 3 to 6 hours. Since nalbuphine is biotransformed by the liver and excreted by the kidney, it should be used at a decreased dosage in patients with hepatic or renal impairment. Although withdrawal reactions have occurred upon rapid cessation of therapy, there are few cases of drug abuse with this compound and, like butorphanol tartrate and dezocine, nalbuphine hydrochloride is not regulated under the Controlled Substances Act.

Oxycodone Hydrochloride. Oxycodone is similar to morphine in its pharmacological effects, except that it is less potent as an analgesic. Although it may be used alone, it is more commonly used in combination with non-opioid analgesics, such as aspirin and acetaminophen and indicated for the reduction of moderate pain.

Oxymorphone Hydrochloride (NUMORPHAN). This drug is a derivative of hydromorphone hydrochloride. Although it is slightly more potent than hydromorphone hydrochloride, the pharmacologic effects and pharmacokinetics are essentially identical.

Pentazocine Lactate (TALWIN). This compound is the oldest of the mixed agonist-antagonist opioids. Its pharmacologic effects are similar to butorphanol tartrate and it produces effective relief of pain predominantly via activity at spinal (kappa receptor) sites. Pentazocine is indicated in the treatment of moderate to moderately severe pain. The cardiovascular effects of this drug differ from the morphine-like compounds, i.e., high doses cause an increase in blood pressure and heart rate; this effect may be the result of an increase in plasma catecholamines observed following the administration of this drug. In addition, psychotomimetic effects, including anxiety, dysphoria, nightmares and hallucinations have been observed, but usually only at the higher dosage levels of the drug. Pentazocine lactate is well absorbed from the gastrointestinal tract; however, first-pass metabolism limits its oral bioavailability to approximately 20 percent. Pentazocine, as the hydrochloride salt, is used by the oral route, but it is combined with naloxone (as TALWIN NX) to reduce the potential for IV use and the abuse of the oral tablets. Dependence can occur with prolonged use, although the incidence is less than with the pure agonist opioids.

Propoxyphene Hydrochloride (DARVON) and Propoxyphene Napsylate (DARVON-N). The analgesic activity of propoxyphene, a derivative of methadone, is found almost entirely in the dextrorotatory isomer, d-propoxyphene (dextropropoxyphene); the levorotatory isomer has significant antitussive activity, but is no longer available for clinical use. Neither salt of propoxyphene (hydrochloride vs. napsylate) offers any advantage over the other. Propoxyphene is a weak analgesic: 65 mg of propoxyphene hydrochloride (or 100 mg of the napsylate salt) is considered no more effective than 650 mg of aspirin or acetaminophen. The drug is only used orally. It is completely absorbed from the gastrointestinal tract, but, due to first-pass biotransformation, the bioavailability is reduced about 50 percent. Propoxyphene is more highly distributed than other opioids (the volume of distribution is between 10 and 20 L/kg) and has a long plasma half-life (approximately 10 hours). The effects of the drug are similar to other opioid analgesics and chronic abuse results in physical dependence.

Sufentanil Citrate (SUFENTA). This compound is used as an IV analgesic adjunct to maintain balanced general anesthesia. It can also be used as a primary anesthetic agent to induce and maintain anesthesia with adequate oxygenation especially in patients undergoing cardiovascular or neurosurgical procedures. It is not indicated for other situations where pain may be present. Sufentanil citrate is between 5 to 10 times more potent than fentanyl. The pharmacologic effects of this drug are very similar to fentanyl and alfentanil; less bradycardia than alfentanil has been reported with this compound. The pharmacokinetics also resemble the two aforementioned drugs. This opioid is biotransformed in the liver and small intestine and excreted by the kidney. Its elimination half-life is 2.7 hr.

NON-OPIOID ANALGESICS

CLASSIFICATION. The non-opioid analgesic drugs (also known as *nonsteroidal anti-inflammatory agents (NSAIDs)* as described above) are a group of structurally-dissimilar organic acids, which are grouped together because they do not bind to opioid receptors. They can be subclassified chemically as outlined in Table 6. This chemical separation has no known clinical importance and is usually made for the convenience of discussion. Although the pharmacologic and toxicologic properties of these compounds are similar and all possess analgesic activity, only certain agents (marked with a * in Table 6) are indicated specifically for the relief of pain.

MECHANISM OF ACTION. Since prostaglandins are formed and released locally in response to cell membrane perturbation, these ubiquitous fatty acid derivatives have become associated with pain reactions that accompany tissue injury and inflammation. Certain prostaglandins, notably PGE_2 and PGI_2 (prostacyclin), sensitize nociceptors of C fibers by lowering the threshold to thermal, mechanical and chemical stimuli. Thus the hyperalgesia induced by prostaglandins is a localized event that allows the mediators of pain, e.g., bradykinin, histamine and substance P, to exert a greater effect on pain receptors.

TABLE 6. SELECTED NON-OPIOID COMPOUNDS

CLASSIFICATION	GENERIC NAME	COMMON TRADE NAMES
Salicylic Acid Derivatives		
	* Aspirin	ECOTRIN, EMPIRIN
	* Diflunisal	DOLOBID
	* Salsalate	DISALCID
	* Choline Magnesium Salicylate	TRILISATE
	* Magnesium Salicylate	MAGAN
	* Sodium Salicylate	
Para-aminophenol Derivative		
	* Acetaminophen	PANADOL, TEMPRA, TYLENOL
Anthranilic Acid Derivatives		
	* Mefenamic Acid	PONSTEL
	* Meclofenamate Sodium	MECLOMEN
Oxicam Derivative		
	Piroxicam	FELDENE
Phenylacetic Acid Derivative		
	Diclofenac Sodium	VOLTAREN
Propionic Acid Derivatives		
	* Fenoprofen Calcium	NALFON
	Flurbiprofen	ANSAID
	* Ibuprofen	ADVIL, MOTRIN, NUPRIN
	* Ketoprofen	ORUDIS
	Nabumetone	RELAFEN
	* Naproxen	NAPROSYN
	* Naproxen Sodium	ANAPROX
	Oxaprozin	DAYPRO
Pyrazolon Derivatives		
	Phenylbutazone	
	Oxyphenbutazone	

TABLE 6 (continued). SELECTED NON-OPIOID COMPOUNDS

CLASSIFICATION	GENERIC NAME	COMMON TRADE NAMES
Indole Derivatives		
	Etodolac	LODINE
	Indomethacin	INDOCIN
	Sulindac	CLINORIL
Pyrrole Derivatives		
	* Ketorolac Tromethamine	TORADOL
	Tolmetin Sodium	TOLECTIN

* Specifically indicated for pain.

All of the non-opioid analgesics prevent the biosynthesis and release of prostaglandins by inhibition of prostaglandin endoperoxide synthase (also called fatty acid cyclooxygenase), a membrane-associated enzyme that is present in almost all cells (see Figure 3). Therefore, the non-opioid analgesics reduce the formation of the prostaglandins, thromboxanes, and prostacyclin, the hyperalgesia caused by these substances, and the pain reactions with which they are associated. As a group, these drugs will not affect the responses of prostaglandins on the tissues; the exception is the anthranilic acid derivatives (fenamates), e.g., mefenamic acid and meclofenamate sodium, which, in addition to inhibiting the endogenous synthesis of the prostaglandins, have been reported to antagonize certain tissue responses of prostaglandins.

Recent studies into the molecular mechanism of these agents show that aspirin (acetylsalicylic acid) acetylates cyclooxygenase, which irreversibly inactivates the enzyme. Other NSAIDs are competitive inhibitors of cyclooxygenase. All NSAIDs studied inhibit both cyclooxygenase-1 (COX-1) and cyclooxygenase-2 (COX-2) to an equal extent.

EFFECTS ON ORGAN SYSTEMS. All of the drugs listed in Table 6 have analgesic, antipyretic, and anti-inflammatory effects; the exception is acetaminophen which lacks clinically-significant anti-inflammatory activity. Not all of the drugs are equally active, nor are all clinically useful, with respect to these effects. Diflunisal, for example, is only weakly antipyretic and is used exclusively as an analgesic. With the exception of acetaminophen, aspirin, and ibuprofen, none of the other compounds are used to reduce fever due to a greater potential for drug toxicity, although most show adequate antipyretic activity.

With the exception of acetaminophen, mefenamic acid, and ketorolac tromethamine, the major use of these drugs is as anti-inflammatory agents in the treatment of various arthritides such as rheumatoid arthritis, ankylosing spondylitis, osteoarthritis, and acute gouty arthritis. As the particular inflammatory condition being treated is alleviated, the pain associated with the disease is also reduced. Therefore, although not specifically indicated as analgesics, pain associated with inflammatory states is effectively reduced by all of these drugs.

Since aspirin is the oldest member of this group of compounds and serves as the prototype to which other compounds are compared, the effects of aspirin on various organ systems will be discussed, with the important differences of the other drugs noted when appropriate.

Gastrointestinal Tract. Localized irritation of the gastrointestinal tract constitutes the most common adverse reaction associated with aspirin and the other drugs in this class. Although epigastric distress is common at the lower dose regimens, gastric and/or intestinal ulceration and bleeding will occur in only a small percentage of patients. At higher doses of aspirin, erosive gastritis and gastrointestinal hemorrhage is observed more often. These effects are the result of inhibition of prostaglandin E_2 and I_2 formation in the gastrointestinal tract; these prostaglandins reduce acid secretion by the stomach and promote the secretion of cytoprotective intestinal mucus. Aspirin and other compounds with high anti-inflammatory activity, e.g., phenylbutazone and indomethacin, tend to elicit the highest incidence of gastrointestinal reactions. Nonacetylated salicylates such as choline magnesium salicylate and magnesium salicylate produce less gastrointestinal problems. Diflunisal and the propionic acid derivatives, fenoprofen calcium, flurbiprofen, ibuprofen, ketoprofen, and naproxen are considered to produce fewer and less intense gastrointestinal reactions than aspirin and are more of a concern in patients with a history of gastrointestinal disorders. Acetaminophen is essentially devoid of these damaging gastrointestinal effects.

Misoprostol (CYTOTEC) reduces the incidence of peptic ulcers when used in conjunction with aspirin or other NSAIDs.

Cardiovascular System. At the usual therapeutic doses employed, none of the non-opioid analgesics have any important effects on the heart or vascular tissues.

Hematologic System. Due to the inhibition of thromboxane A_2 formation in thrombocytes, reduced platelet aggregation and prolonged bleeding time may occur with aspirin and the effect is considered to be "irreversible", i.e., it persists for the life of the platelet. For example, mean bleeding time in a normal patient will be doubled for 4 to 7 days following the ingestion of 650 mg of aspirin. All of the other non-opioid analgesics, except acetaminophen, will inhibit platelet aggregation, however the effect is "reversible", usually quantitatively less and of shorter duration than that observed with aspirin. Increased bleeding time may become exacerbated in persons with underlying hematologic defects or in patients on anticoagulant therapy, and the use of any NSAID in these individuals should be with caution and awareness of the potential problem.

Renal System. Sodium and water retention with edema constitute potential adverse effects of these drugs; however, with the exception of phenylbutazone these effects are uncommon and not a significant clinical problem. Nephrotoxicity, manifested as acute interstitial nephritis with hematuria, proteinuria, and the nephrotic syndrome, although rarely observed, has been reported in patients taking aspirin or several of the other NSAIDs for a prolonged period of time.

Many of the compounds in this group have weak uricosuric activity, but are not useful for this purpose. Aspirin, in doses below 2 g per day, may reduce urate excretion and elevate plasma urate levels, while large doses, i.e., over 5 g per day, induce uricosuria and lower the plasma urate concentration. Since these large doses of aspirin are poorly tolerated and more potent, less toxic uricosurics, e.g., probenecid (BENEMID) and sulfinpyrazone (ANTURANE), are available, aspirin should not be considered as a useful uricosuric. Furthermore, in patients with hyperuricemia, small analgesic doses of aspirin will reduce the effectiveness of both probenecid and sulfinpyrazone and may precipitate an attack of gout. The mechanisms responsible for this drug-drug interaction are complex and beyond the scope of this book.

Respiratory System and Acid-Base Balance. Small analgesic doses of aspirin, e.g., 325 to 650 mg, resulting in plasma salicylate concentrations of 50 to 100 μg/mL do not affect respiration; larger doses increase metabolic oxygen consumption and carbon dioxide (CO_2) production which stimulates respiration. Plasma CO_2 tension initially does not increase since respiratory stimulation (mainly depth of respiration) enhances CO_2 elimination. At higher plasma salicylate concentrations (approximately 350 μg/mL), direct stimulation of the medullary respiratory center occurs; this results in hyperventilation and respiratory alkalosis as CO_2 loss increases. Compensation for the respiratory alkalosis occurs via enhanced renal excretion of sodium, potassium, and bicarbonate which normalizes blood pH. Adults compensate quite well to changes in respiration and acid-base balance and rarely do these effects progress beyond this point. Occasionally, adults may develop more severe problems following large doses of salicylates; more commonly, children, because of their smaller body weight, present with acute salicylate toxicity.

Respiratory paralysis will be observed at a plasma salicylate concentration above 460 μg/mL due to drug-induced depression of the medulla. Since enhanced CO_2 production continues, respiratory and metabolic acidosis ensues and circulatory collapse, secondary to vasomotor depression, will follow. Increased renal excretion of bicarbonate decreases the plasma bicarbonate concentration and, therefore, the respiratory acidosis is uncompensated. Furthermore, metabolic acidosis exacerbates the condition due to the large concentration of salicylate (an acid) in the blood and the accumulation of organic acids, e.g., pyruvic, lactic and acetoacetic acids, due to salicylate-induced alterations in carbohydrate metabolism. Treatment for the acidosis involves the intravenous infusion of sodium bicarbonate.

In contrast to aspirin, none of the other drugs in this category have been associated with clinically-significant alterations in respiratory function or acid-base balance.

Hepatic System. Salicylates, including aspirin have been reported to cause mild hepatotoxicity. More severe problems may occur in patients with a history of chronic liver disease. Other NSAIDs rarely produce severe hepatotoxicity. However, acetaminophen may produce fatal hepatotoxicity, in overdose, due to production of an hepatotoxic metabolite.

Hypersensitivity. NSAIDs have been reported to produce cutaneous hypersensitivity reactions, e.g., urticaria, photosensitivity, or pruritus. Aspirin and other NSAIDs may also produce a nonimmunologic response resulting in bronchospasm and rhinitis or angioedema and urticaria.

Central Nervous System. Aspirin and the other non-opioid analgesics may induce a mild adverse syndrome known as *salicylism*. Part of the symptom complex involves the central nervous system and includes headache, dizziness, tinnitus, mental confusion, drowsiness, lassitude and decreased visual and auditory acuity. In the more severe cases, generalized convulsions may be observed. Although salicylism is commonly associated with the salicylates, most of the other non-opioid analgesics have been reported to produce these effects.

PHARMACOKINETICS. A comparisons of the some of the pharmacokinetic data for these drugs are shown in Table 7. All of the non-opioid analgesics are well absorbed following oral administration; the oral bioavailability ranges from 50 to 100 percent. The analgesic effect has an onset within 0.5 to 1 hour and peaks within 3 to 4 hours for all of these drugs. Depending on the compound, the duration of analgesic activity may be up to 12 hours, especially during chronic administration, since the plasma elimination half-life of these drugs is dose-dependent and tends to be longer at steady-state plasma levels. All of the drugs distribute throughout most body tissues and fluids but have a relatively low apparent volume of distribution due to high plasma protein binding; the major exception is acetaminophen which is not highly protein bound and distributes more completely. Although a few compounds may be biotransformed to active derivatives, e.g., aspirin to salicylic acid and phenylbutazone to oxyphenbutazone, in general, hepatic biotransformation to inactive oxidized and conjugated products precedes the elimination of these drugs, primarily in the urine. Some compounds, e.g., diclofenac sodium, may also be excreted through the bile. Sulindac is

TABLE 7. PHARMACOKINETIC DATA OF NON-OPIOID ANALGESICS

DRUG NAMES GENERIC AND (TRADE)	ORAL BIOAVAILABILITY (Percent)	TIME TO PEAK PLASMA CONC. (Hours)	ELIMINATION HALF-LIFE (Hours)	PLASMA PROTEIN BINDING (Percent)	VOLUME OF DISTRIBUTION (L/kg)	EFFECTIVE PLASMA CONCENTRATIONS (μg/mL)
Acetaminophen (TYLENOL, etc.)	90 to 100	0.5 to 1	2	20	0.80 to 1.00	10 to 20
Aspirin (ECOTRIN, EMPIRIN, etc.)	65 to 70	0.5 to 1	0.25 to 0.35[a]	80 to 90	0.15 to 0.20	20
Salicylic Acid	95 to 100	------------[b]	2 to 3[a]	80 to 90	0.13 to 0.17	50 to 100
Diclofenac Sodium (VOLTAREN)	45 to 55	2 to 3	2	99	0.50 to 0.60	1 to 2
Diflunisal (DOLOBID)	90 to 100	2 to 3	8 to 12[a]	99	0.08 to 0.10	------------
Etodolac (LODINE)	80 to 90	1 to 2	7 to 8	99	------------	------------
Fenoprofen Calcium (NALFON)	85 to 90	1 to 2	3	99	0.08 to 0.10	25 to 50
Flurbiprofen (ANSAID)	90 to 100	1 to 2	3 to 9	99	------------	10 to 20
Ibuprofen (ADVIL, MOTRIN, NUPRIN, etc.)	80 to 90	0.5 to 1.5	2	95 to 99	0.15 to 0.17	------------
Indomethacin (INDOCIN)	95 to 98	2	2 to 3	90	0.25 to 0.30	0.3 to 1.0
Ketorolac Tromethamine (TORADOL)	99 to 100	0.5 to 0.6	4 to 6	99	0.15 to 0.33	------------
Meclofenamate Sodium (MECLOMEN)	------------	0.5 to 1	2	99	------------	------------
Mefenamic Acid (PONSTEL)	------------	2 to 4	2	99	------------	------------
Nabumetone (RELAFEN)	80 to 100	3	24	99	0.7	------------
Naproxen (NAPROSYN)	95 to 100	2 to 4	13 to 15	99	0.15 to 0.17	25 to 50
Naproxen Sodium (ANAPROX)	95 to 100	2 to 4	13 to 15	99	0.15 to 0.17	25 to 50
Oxaprozin (DAYPRO)	90 to 100	3 to 5	50	99	------------	------------
Phenylbutazone	80 to 100	1 to 3	60 100	98	0.09 to 0.10	50 to 150
Piroxicam (FELDENE)	90 to 100	3 to 5	30 to 80	99	0.12 to 0.14	1.5 to 2
Sulindac (CLINORIL)	85 to 95	2	7 to 18	90 to 95	------------	------------
Tolmetin Sodium (TOLECTIN)	90 to 100	0.5 to 1	1 to 2	99	0.09 to 0.12	------------

[a] The elimination kinetics of salicylates are complex since some of the enzymes involved in the biotransformation of salicylates are saturable at therapeutic plasma concentrations. Therefore, the elimination half-life increases with dose, e.g., with salicylic acid: at 325 to 650 mg (administered as aspirin) the elimination half-life is 2 - 3 hours; at 1000 mg, it is 5 - 8 hours; and at 2000 mg, it is 8 - 16 hours.

[b] ------------ indicates that no data are available.

interesting since it is an inactive compound, biotransformed in the liver by oxidation to the inactive sulfone and by reduction to the sulfide, the active moiety.

DRUG MONOGRAPHS. The following drug monographs contain supplemental information concerning each of the non-opioid analgesics listed above. Following the monograph on aspirin, the prototype of the non-opioid analgesics, monographs on the other non-opioid analgesics are arranged alphabetically by the generic name of the drug. Representative pharmaceutical preparations that are available, common adult and pediatric doses, and routes of administration are listed in Table H (pp. 124 - 134), Table I (pp. 135 - 137), Table J (p. 138), and Table K (pp. 140 - 143).

Aspirin (BAYER ASPIRIN, EMPIRIN, others). Although aspirin (acetylsalicylic acid) is the oldest member of this class of drugs, it remains as a drug of choice for mild to moderate analgesic conditions including headache, myalgia, and arthralgia. The pharmacologic effects of aspirin are described above and supplementation is not necessary here. It is important to mention that the use of aspirin as an analgesic or antipyretic in children has come under scrutiny due to the association of the drug in treating varicella (chicken pox) or influenza virus infections and the development of Reye's syndrome. Consequently, if fever, headache, etc., are present in children and either of these viruses is suspected, aspirin should not be prescribed for children or teenagers and alternative measures, e.g., acetaminophen or ibuprofen, should be used. Some of the pharmacokinetics of aspirin are shown in Table 7 along with those of salicylic acid, the active biotransformation product and the major circulating salicylate following aspirin administration. The bioavailability of aspirin itself is one of the lowest of the NSAIDs, but since some of the drug is hydrolyzed to salicylic acid in the stomach, oral absorption of aspirin is actually rather complete. Food slows the absorption of aspirin and the bioavailability of enteric coated preparations (e.g., BAYER ENTERIC ASPIRIN, ECOTRIN), used to reduce gastric intolerance, may be erratic. Aspirin rectal suppositories are available for patients who cannot use the oral preparations; absorption by this route is slow and incomplete and rectal mucosal irritation may occur. Other salicylates are discussed below.

Acetaminophen (PANADOL, TEMPRA, TYLENOL, others). Acetaminophen is a well-tolerated analgesic and antipyretic drug that lacks significant anti-inflammatory activity. The analgesic potency is identical to aspirin and like aspirin, acetaminophen is used alone to treat milder analgesic situations and may be combined with an opioid analgesic for moderate to severe pain reactions. The drug is especially of value in patients who are allergic to aspirin, have hemostatic disturbances or are taking anticoagulant drugs, have gastric ulcers or gastritis, or are being treated for gouty arthritis, since acetaminophen does not affect bleeding time, cause gastrointestinal upset, or modify sodium urate excretion. Adverse reactions to the compound occur infrequently, but may include allergic reactions such as skin rashes and drug-related fever. Hepatic toxicity may occur following the acute administration of large doses of the drug (10 to 15 g) and larger amounts (25 g or more) are potentially fatal. The hepatic necrosis that has been observed is due to the formation of N-acetyl-benzoquinoneimine, a highly-reactive intermediate, which reacts with glutathione and sulfhydryl groups in proteins. The treatment for this drug toxicity involves the oral use of acetylcysteine (MUCOMYST), which binds the offending metabolite and spares the liver. The pharmacokinetics of acetaminophen are similar to the salicylates, except that plasma protein binding is low. Consequently, the volume of distribution of this drug is greater and drug-drug interactions involving competition for plasma protein binding sites are insignificant. Acetaminophen is widely used orally; however, rectal suppositories are available and are useful especially in children for treatment of pain and fever.

Diclofenac Sodium (VOLTAREN). Diclofenac sodium has all of the pharmacological properties attributed to NSAIDs. At present, by oral administration, it is only indicated for the treatment of inflammatory states, i.e., rheumatoid arthritis, osteoarthritis, and ankylosing spondylitis; an ophthalmic solution is available for the treatment of postoperative inflammation after cataract extraction. Although almost completely absorbed from the gastrointestinal tract following oral administration, the oral bioavailability is low (approximately 50 percent) due to high first-pass metabolism to mono- and di-hydroxylated products. Diclofenac sodium is highly bound to plasma proteins; however, in comparison to other NSAIDs it appears to have a high volume of distribution. Approximately 65 percent of an oral dose is eliminated in the urine, 35 percent via the bile as inactive biotransformation products.

Diflunisal (DOLOBID). This compound is a difluorophenyl derivative of salicylic acid which has significant analgesic and anti-inflammatory activity, but is only weakly antipyretic and therefore not used for fever. Similar to other salicylate derivatives, diflunisal is well absorbed following oral administration, is highly bound to plasma proteins, and is excreted in the urine mainly as inactive glucuronides. It has a longer plasma half-life than aspirin (see Table 7) and is not biotransformed to salicylic acid *in vivo*. In terms of potency and analgesic efficacy, 500 mg of diflunisal is comparable to 650 mg of aspirin.

Etodolac (LODINE). Etodolac, like other NSAIDs, acts through inhibition of prostaglandin synthesis. It has anti-inflammatory, analgesic, and antipyretic activity. The drug is specifically indicated for the management of osteoarthritis. It may also be used for relief of general pain. Etodolac is as effective in the therapy of osteoarthritis as aspirin, diclofenac, or piroxicam. Adverse reactions are similar to other NSAIDs, the most common of which is gastrointestinal distress, including dyspepsia, abdominal pain, diarrhea, and nausea. Other adverse reactions, reported in greater than 3 percent of patients, include malaise and dizziness. Slight elevations in liver enzymes may occur. The drug is well absorbed from the gastrointestinal tract and approximately 70 percent of the administered dose is eliminated in the urine, mostly as metabolic products.

Fenoprofen Calcium (NALFON). Fenoprofen calcium is a typical non-opioid analgesic, anti-inflammatory, and antipyretic compound. In terms of analgesic efficacy, 200 mg of fenoprofen calcium is equal to 650 mg of aspirin. Its pharmacokinetics are unremarkable and except for possibly less gastrointestinal complaints, the drug offers no advantage over other analgesic agents in this class.

Flurbiprofen (ANSAID). This fluorinated propionic acid derivative has pharmacologic effects that are typical of other drugs in this class. At this time, oral flurbiprofen is indicated only for the acute or long-term treatment of symptoms of rheumatoid arthritis and osteoarthritis; a topical preparation (OCUFEN) has recently been approved for inhibition of intraoperative miosis. Similar to most NSAIDs, this drug is well absorbed following oral administration and reaches a peak plasma concentration in 1 to 2 hours. The elimination half-life of flurbiprofen is about 6 hours; the drug is extensively biotransformed in the liver (predominantly to inactive hydroxylated products) and excreted in the urine.

Ibuprofen (ADVIL, MOTRIN, NUPRIN, others). Ibuprofen was the first of the propionic acid derivatives to be used clinically and has found utility as an analgesic, antipyretic, and anti-inflammatory agent. Caplets and tablets containing 200 mg of ibuprofen are available over-the-counter for the temporary relief of minor pains and for the reduction of fever (see Table H), although 400 mg is considered a proper analgesic dose for moderate pain. At 200 to 400 mg, the drug is effective for the pain of primary dysmenorrhea, and daily amounts of up to 3200 mg in divided doses may be used for rheumatoid arthritis and osteoarthritis. In general, the incidence of adverse effects with ibuprofen is low; the most common problems are gastrointestinal complaints. Other common adverse reactions include dizziness, headache, rashes, and tinnitus. In comparison to 650 mg of aspirin, an equianalgesic dose of ibuprofen (200 to 400 mg) appears to induce less gastric erosion than the protype salicylate.

Indomethacin (INDOCIN). This compound is one of the most potent of the nonsteroidal anti-inflammatory agents and is used to treat moderate to severe inflammatory conditions; it is not recommended for use as an analgesic or an antipyretic. Generally the compound is used by the oral route, but rectal suppositories are available for patients who cannot tolerate the oral dosage forms. In addition, indomethacin sodium trihydrate administered intravenously, is indicated for the closure of a patent ductus arteriosus in premature infants. The most common adverse reactions include gastrointestinal irritation, nausea, anorexia, abdominal pain, headache, dizziness, and mental confusion. Indomethacin does not alter the uricosuric activity of probenecid and apparently does not affect bleeding time or enhance the activity of the oral anticoagulants. It has been shown to antagonize the diuresis induced by furosemide and the antihypertensive effects of thiazide diuretics and β-adrenergic blocking agents.

Ketoprofen (ORUDIS). Ketoprofen is a relatively new propionic acid derivative. Its pharmacological and toxicological activity is similar to other NSAIDs and rather unremarkable. Clinical studies have shown the drug to be comparable to other NSAIDs in the treatment of mild to moderate pain of unknown origin and the pain associated with rheumatoid arthritis, ankylosing spondylitis, and acute gout; in comparison to aspirin, the incidence of gastrointestinal complaints is low.

Ketorolac Tromethamine (TORADOL). Ketorolac is a substituted pyrrole derivative that is structurally related to tolmetin. Like most other non-opioid analgesics, ketorolac acts by inhibition of prostaglandin synthesis and has analgesic, anti-inflammatory and antipyretic activities; however, it appears that the analgesic activity of this compound is greater than its anti-inflammatory potency. The marketed product, i.e., TORADOL, is unique in that it is the only drug of this type available for intramuscular (IM) as well as oral administration for the short-term management of moderate to severe pain; clinical studies indicate that this drug is at least as effective, if not superior to morphine, meperidine, or pentazocine for the treatment of moderate to severe postoperative pain. Ketorolac tromethamine is completely absorbed following IM administration; mean peak plasma concentrations of 2.2 to 3.0 μg/mL occur within 1 hour after a single 30 mg dose. Similar to most other non-opioid analgesics, ketorolac tromethamine is highly bound to plasma proteins resulting in a low apparent volume of distribution (see Table 7). The drug is biotransformed by hydroxylation and conjugation reactions in the liver and most of the parent compound and the metabolites and eliminated in the urine. The mean elimination half-life has been calculated to be 4.5 hours in young adults and 7.0 hours in the elderly. Adverse reactions, warnings, precautions, and contraindications of ketorolac tromethamine are similar to other non-opioid analgesics.

Ketorolac tromethamine has recently been approved for use as an ophthalmic solution (ACULAR) to relieve ocular itching in seasonal allergic conjunctivitis. It has been shown to reduce prostaglandin concentrations in the eye, which are believed to be associated with the itching.

Meclofenamate Sodium (MECLOMEN). This compound is an anthranilic acid derivative, chemically related to mefenamic acid. It appears to be a more potent anti-inflammatory compound than mefenamic acid and is used for this purpose (rheumatoid arthritis and osteoarthritis) as well as for mild to moderate pain. The incidence of mild adverse reactions such as those typically associated with other NSAIDs is high (and thus the compound is not a drug of first choice); however, the severe hematologic abnormalities commonly associated with mefenamic acid are less prevalent with meclofenamate sodium. This drug is biotransformed partially to a hydroxymethyl derivative (which also has anti-inflammatory activity) and an inactive carboxyl derivative, both of which are conjugated with glucuronic acid prior to elimination. Approximately 65 percent of the drug and its metabolites are excreted in the urine, and the remainder in the feces.

Mefenamic Acid (PONSTEL). Mefenamic acid has a number of potentially severe adverse effects which limit its usefulness. In addition to a myriad of gastrointestinal problems, patients may experience dizziness, drowsiness, headache, blurred vision, rashes, and facial edema. More importantly, the drug has caused decreased hematocrit, leukopenia, eosinophilia, agranulocytosis, and pancytopenia. Although mefenamic acid is an effective analgesic and is indicated for the relief of moderate pain and for primary dysmenorrhea, therapy with this drug should not exceed one week.

Nabumetone (RELAFEN). Nabumetone is an NSAID exhibiting anti-inflammatory, analgesic, and antipyretic properties. It is specifically indicated for both acute and chronic management of osteoarthritis and rheumatoid arthritis. The compound is a prodrug, with approximately 35 percent biotransformed in the liver to 6-methoxy-2-naphthylacetic acid (MNA), a potent inhibitor of cyclooxygenase; 50 percent is metabolized to other products. MNA, the active metabolite, is highly bound to plasma proteins (over 99 percent). The most frequent adverse reaction to this drug is gastrointestinal distress including diarrhea, dyspepsia, and abdominal pain. Other reactions are similar to other NSAIDs and may include dizziness, headache, pruritus, rash, tinnitus, and edema.

Naproxen (NAPROSYN) and Naproxen Sodium (ANAPROX). These two drugs have identical pharmacologic activity and therapeutic uses. The only difference is that the sodium salt is more rapidly absorbed following oral administration and produces higher peak plasma levels than naproxen itself. The activity of the compound is terminated predominantly by glucuronide conjugation, although approximately 30 percent of the drug may be converted to an inactive methylated product. Interestingly, the biotransformation is slower than most of the other non-opioid analgesics, resulting in a longer plasma half-life for naproxen, i.e., 13 to 15 hours. Therefore, this drug can be used on a twice a day basis. In addition to the use of naproxen for rheumatoid arthritis, gout, osteoarthritis, and ankylosing spondylitis, the compound has been found to be effective for mild to moderate pain and for the treatment of primary dysmenorrhea.

Oxaprozin (DAYPRO). Oxaprozin is a propionic acid derivative with analgesic, anti-inflammatory, and antipyretic activity. Like other NSAIDs, the drug is an inhibitor of cyclooxygenase. It is useful in the management of osteoarthritis and rheumatoid arthritis. The most common adverse reactions are similar to those reported for other NSAIDs. Oxaprozin has greater than 95 percent oral bioavailability and is highly bound to plasma proteins. The drug is removed from the plasma primarily by hepatic metabolism; a glucuronide metabolite is secreted into the bile and eliminated in the feces. Oxaprozin has a long elimination half-life due to low hepatic and renal clearance.

Phenylbutazone. Phenylbutazone has all of the effects associated with the other NSAIDs; however, because of its toxicity it should not be used for pain or reduction of fever. Common adverse reactions of phenylbutazone include gastrointestinal disturbances, sodium and water retention with edema, and rashes. The drug has also caused hepatic and renal tubular necrosis, the nephrotic syndrome, optic neuritis, and deafness. The most serious adverse effects of this drug are blood dyscrasias including leukopenia, pancytopenia, agranulocytosis, and aplastic anemia; since these are rare if the drug is used for short periods of time, the use of phenylbutazone as an anti-inflammatory agent should be restricted to 7 days in duration. Phenylbutazone is partially biotransformed to an active hydroxylated product, oxyphenbutazone, which has the same pharmacology as the parent drug. Both compounds are highly and tightly bound to plasma proteins, resulting in long plasma half-lives (60 to 100 hours for phenylbutazone, 55 to 90 hours for oxyphenbutazone); therapeutically, however, phenylbutazone must be administered 4 times daily to maintain an effective free plasma concentration of the drug.

Piroxicam (FELDENE). This compound is structurally dissimilar from all other non-opioid analgesics; however, it has pharmacologic properties common to the group. Although a few studies have shown that piroxicam is effective for the relief of postoperative pain, dental pain, and the pain of traumas, at present it is only indicated for the treatment of inflammatory conditions. The drug is extensively biotransformed to inactive products; however, enterohepatic recirculation of the parent drug results in a long plasma half-life (approximately 50 hours) and the ability to use this drug once per day. Adverse reactions are similar to most of the others NSAIDs; severe hematologic problems have only rarely been observed.

Salicylates. In addition to aspirin and diflunisal, other salicylates are available for use as anti-inflammatory or analgesic agents. The topical administration of salicylic acid (for keratolysis in the treatment of acne or corns) and methylsalicylate (as a counterirritant for sore muscles) will not be considered.

Salsalate (DISALCID) is salicylsalicylic acid, a dimer of salicylic acid. This compound is quite insoluble in the acidic gastric fluid, but readily dissolves in the alkaline environment of the small intestine. Some of the drug is hydrolyzed to salicylic acid in the intestinal lumen following oral administration; however, most is absorbed unchanged. In the plasma, rapid hydrolysis to the active moiety, salicylic acid, occurs via plasma esterases. Thus salsalate is another way of achieving analgesic/anti-inflammatory plasma salicylate levels. Most of the pharmacologic effects of this drug are identical to those of aspirin. In contrast to aspirin, salsalate does not cause a significant inhibition of platelet aggregation and the incidence of gastrointestinal upset appears to be less than equi-effective doses of aspirin.

Salicylic acid itself is very irritating to the gastrointestinal mucosa; therefore, this compound is never used systemically. Sodium salicylate is available for oral administration as an analgesic, but it is less effective than equal doses of aspirin and is rarely used due to a high incidence of gastrointestinal upset. Magnesium salicylate (MAGAN) is used for pain and choline magnesium salicylate (TRILISATE) is used for pain and, of occasion, for the treatment of osteoarthritis, rheumatoid arthritis, and other arthritides.

Sulindac (CLINORIL). Sulindac is a structural derivative of indomethacin and has similar pharmacologic and toxicologic activity. It is considered to be a prodrug since it is inactive; in the liver it is converted to sulindac sulfide, the active biotransformation product. Sulindac and its sulfide metabolite are excreted in the bile and reabsorbed in the intestine; the long half-life of the drug is due to this enterohepatic recirculation. The drug is an effective anti-inflammatory agent and useful for the pain associated with conditions such as osteoarthritis, rheumatoid arthritis and bursitis.

Tolmetin Sodium (TOLECTIN). The pharmacologic activity of tolmetin sodium is similar in most respects to indomethacin and sulindac. Similar to these two drugs, tolmetin is indicated for inflammatory states and is not recommended for the treatment of non-inflammatory pain. This compound differs from indomethacin and sulindac only in that it does not appear to produce clinically-significant changes in platelet aggregation, and although it binds to a high degree to plasma proteins, tolmetin does not alter therapy with oral anticoagulants or hypoglycemics.

REFERENCES

------- "General Analgesics," In: *Drug Evaluations Annual 1993*, American Medical Association, Chicago, 1993, pp. 169-190.

------- "Antiarthritic Drugs," In: *Drug Evaluations Annual 1993*, American Medical Association, Chicago, 1993, pp. 1889-1934.

------- "Drugs for Pain," In: *The Medical Letter* **35 (Issue 887)**: 1-6 (1993).

Buckley, M.M.-T., and R.N. Brogden: "Ketorolac: A Review of its Pharmacodynamic and Pharmacokinetic Properties, and Therapeutic Potential," *Drugs* **39**: 86-109 (1990).

Cohen, L.S.: "Clinical Pharmacology of Acetylsalicylic Acid," *Seminar. Thromb. Hemostas.* **2**: 146-175 (1976).

Dickenson, A.H.: "Mechanism of the Analgesic Actions of Opiates and Opioids", *Brit. Med. J.* **47**: 691-702 (1991).

Flower, R.J.: "Drugs Which Inhibit Prostaglandin Biosynthesis," *Pharmacol. Rev.* **26**: 33-67 (1974).

Insel, P.A.: "Analgesic-Antipyretics and Anti-inflammatory Agents," In: *The Pharmacological Basis of Therapeutics, Eighth Edition*, Gilman, A.G., T.W. Rall, A.S. Nies, and P. Taylor (Eds.), Pergamon Press, New York, 1990, pp. 638-670.

Jaffe, J.H., and W.R. Martin, W.R.: "Opioid Analgesics and Antagonists," In: *The Pharmacological Basis of Therapeutics, Eighth Edition*, Gilman, A.G., T.W. Rall, A.S. Nies, and P. Taylor (Eds.), Pergamon Press, New York, 1990, pp. 485-521.

Klepstad, P., A. Maurset, L.E.R. Moberg, and I. Oye: "Evidence of a Role for NMDA Receptors in Pain Perception," *Eur. J. Pharmacol.* **187**: 513-518 (1990).

Loh, H.H., and A.P. Smith: "Molecular Characterization of Opioid Receptors," *Annu. Rev. Pharmacol.* **30**: 123-147 (1990).

Martin, W.R.: "Pharmacology of Opioids," *Pharmacol. Rev.* **35**: 283-322 (1983).

Monk, J.P., R. Beresford, and A. Ward: "Sufentanil. A Review of its Pharmacological Properties and Therapeutic Use," *Drugs* **36**: 286-313 (1988).

Nakajima, Y., S. Nakajima, M. and Inque: "Substance P Induced Inhibition of Potassium Channels via a Pertussin Toxin-Insensitive G Protein," In: *Substance P and Related Peptides: Cellular and Molecular Physiology*, Leeman, S.E., J.E. Krause, and F. Lelmbeck (Eds.), *Ann. N.Y. Acad. Sci.* **632**: 103-111 (1991).

Nickander, R., F.G. McMahon, and A.S. Ridolfo: "Non-steroidal Anti-inflammatory Agents", *Annu. Rev. Pharmacol. Toxicol.* **19**: 469-490 (1979).

Pastenak, G.W.: "Pharmacological Mechanisms of Opioid Analgesics," *Clin. Neuropharmacol.* **16**: 1-18 (1993).

Rowland, M. and S. Riegelman: "Pharmacokinetics of Acetylsalicylic Acid and Salicylic Acid After Intravenous Administration in Man," *J. Pharm. Sci.* **57**: 1313-1319 (1968).

Walker, J.M., W.D. Bowen, F.O. Walker, R.R. Matsumoto, B. deCosta, and K.C. Rice: "Sigma Receptors: Biology and Function," *Pharmacol. Rev.* **42**: 355-402 (1990).

Wilcox, G.L.: "Excitatory Neurotransmitters and Pain," In: *Proceedings of the VIth World Congress on Pain, Chapter 12*, Bond, M.R., J.E. Charlton, and C.F. Woolf (Eds.), Elsevier, New York, 1991.

MANAGEMENT

OF

PAIN

CLINICAL APPROACH TO PAIN CONTROL

In order to fulfill one of the primary responsibilities of medicine, the physician is faced with the task of choosing appropriate methods for the management of pain. The approach taken is often variable, depending on the underlying nature of the responsible disease process. The use of potent opioids may be the course taken in one circumstance, however, this approach may be completely inappropriate in another. The physician may have to settle for less than complete pain relief in the short term in order to avoid long-term drug complications. Pain experienced by patients can be subdivided into two main types: acute and chronic (or frequently recurring). An approach to the management of these specific pain syndromes is discussed below and is summarized in Table 8.

ACUTE PAIN

Acute pain is usually self-limiting, and from a therapeutic point of view, can be subdivided on the basis of intensity, e.g., mild, moderate and severe. For the sake of discussion, acute pain will be divided into only two degrees, i.e., mild to moderate, and severe.

THERAPY OF MILD TO MODERATE PAIN. Mild to moderate pain usually originates from a variety of minor traumas or localized inflammatory processes of ligaments, muscles, bones, and joints. Initially, this type of pain is best managed with 650 to 1000 mg of either aspirin (plain or buffered) or acetaminophen every 4 hours orally. If the pain is associated with a large inflammatory component, such as that resulting from a torn ligament, aspirin would be preferred since acetaminophen lacks significant anti-inflammatory activity. For those patients who prefer to take medications less often, or for those with inflammatory pain and gastrointestinal intolerance to aspirin, the standard doses of any of the other non-opioid analgesics (also known as *nonsteroidal anti-inflammatory drugs* or *NSAIDs*), except phenylbutazone, oxyphenbutazone, or indomethacin (INDOCIN), may be used as the initial therapy (see Table H for drugs, available preparations and common dosages). Most of these drugs are used every 6 to 8 hours; sulindac (CLINORIL) and diflunisal (DOLOBID) may be used every 12 hours and nabumetone (RELAFEN), oxaprozin (DAYPRO), and piroxicam (FELDENE) may be used once daily. It should be noted that only ibuprofen (ADVIL, MOTRIN, NUPRIN, etc.),

TABLE 8. A STEPWISE APPROACH TO PAIN MANAGEMENT FOR SPECIFIC SYNDROMES

TYPE OF PAIN	INITIAL REGIMEN	IF RESPONSE IS INADEQUATE	IF RESPONSE IS STILL INADEQUATE
ACUTE PAIN			
Mild to moderate	Acetaminophen, aspirin or another NSAID	Add codeine, oxycodone, propoxyphene or pentazocine orally	Reevaluate the cause(s) of the pain
Severe	Parenteral opioids	Add parenteral hydroxyzine; increase the opioid dose, or add an NSAID if the patient can take oral medications; consider using a tricyclic antidepressant	Reevaluate the cause(s) of the pain
CHRONIC PAIN			
Benign	Acetaminophen, aspirin or another NSAID	Add analgesic adjuvants, or use an oral mixed agonist-antagonist opioid agent as infrequently as possible	Consider a neurosurgical or anesthetic procedure
Terminal, cancer related	Acetaminophen, aspirin or another NSAID with or without oxycodone, codeine, propoxyphene or pentazocine	Substitute oral morphine, hydromorphone, methadone or meperidine for the other oral opioid, or may consider use of fentanyl transdermal	Add parenteral opioids, epidural or intrathecal opioid infusion, or analgesic adjuvants

NSAID = nonsteroidal anti-inflammatory drug

ketoprofen (ORUDIS), diflunisal (DOLOBID), etodolac (LODINE), fenoprofen calcium (NALFON), naproxen (NAPROSYN), naproxen sodium (ANAPROX), mefenamic acid (PONSTEL) and meclofenamate sodium (MECLOMEN) are specifically indicated in their product information for the management of mild to moderate pain. In addition there are several studies documenting the effectiveness of NSAIDs in inflammatory pain, when compared to opioids. For example, studies have shown that a dose of 400 to 800 mg of ibuprofen (MOTRIN) is as effective as 30 to 60 mg of codeine and is more effective than 65 mg of propoxyphene hydrochloride (DARVON).

If an inadequate therapeutic response occurs with the non-opioid agents, then the addition of a low potency oral opioid compound (see Table D) to the pain regimen may be appropriate. Codeine sulfate or phosphate, 30 to 60 mg; oxycodone hydrochloride, 5 to 10 mg; propoxyphene hydrochloride (DARVON), 65 mg; propoxyphene napsylate (DARVON-N), 100 mg; or pentazocine hydrochloride (TALWIN NX), 50 mg, every 4 to 6 hours are commonly employed for this purpose. In general, analgesia resulting from these agents will be additive to that produced by the non-opioids, since both classes of compounds act through different mechanisms and are complementary in their effects. Each of these opioid analgesics has its own particular advantages and disadvantages, and the choice of a given agent is usually governed by the prescribing habits of the physician and the past experience of the patient. In general, codeine seems to be the most constipating, oxycodone has the fastest onset of action (but may also have a higher abuse potential), propoxyphene is the least potent (but nonetheless abuse potential is definitely present), and pentazocine, being an agonist-antagonist, appears to have a lower abuse potential but a higher incidence of psychotomimetic effects.

To exploit the additive effects of opioid and non-opioid analgesics, several pharmaceutical companies offer fixed-dose combinations of these drugs (see Table K). Although it may be more convenient to prescribe these combination products, problems can result from both the patient and physician not understanding the exact composition and dosages of the medications contained within these formulations. Also, these fixed-dose combinations do not allow much freedom in titrating one component upward while keeping the other component constant.

THERAPY OF SEVERE PAIN. Severe pain, such as that following surgery or major trauma, usually requires the use of potent parenteral opioids (see Table D). With the exception of alfentanil hydrochloride (ALFENTA), fentanyl citrate (SUBLIMAZE), and sufentanil citrate (SUFENTA), which are used during surgery, any one of the agonist or agonist-antagonist agents could be administered, provided a sufficient amount is given to relieve pain without causing severe adverse effects. The key to proper pain management in this setting is individualization of the dose of the particular opioid based on the needs of the patient. Because of significant differences in body weight, obese patients have a higher opioid requirement than emaciated patients. Elderly patients, because of altered drug disposition and receptor sensitivity, usually require a smaller opioid dose than their younger counterparts. The use of analgesic adjuvants, e.g., hydroxyzine (ATARAX, VISTARIL), the benzodiazepines, tricyclic antidepessants, etc., may also have a role in the management of severe acute pain (see pp. 68 - 71).

One of the most common misconceptions among physicians and other health care personnel is that the short term use of large doses of parenteral opioids for acute pain could make the patient physically dependent on these drugs. However, it generally takes at least ten days of exposure to moderate doses of opioids before the patient will begin to exhibit signs of tolerance or physical dependence. In addition, the availability of parenteral opioids with agonist-antagonist properties and reduced dependence liabilities, e.g., butorphanol tartrate (STADOL), nalbuphine hydrochloride (NUBAIN), dezocine (DALGAN), and buprenorphine hydrochloride (BUPRENEX), should free the physician from worrying about physical dependence when using opioids acutely. Ketorolac tromethamine (TORADOL), a parenteral, as well as an oral, non-opioid analgesic, has been marketed for use in moderate to severe post-operative pain. Clinical studies have shown that the efficacy of single doses of this drug is equal to or greater than morphine, meperidine, or pentazocine; furthermore, the drug has not been observed to cause either physical or psychologic drug dependence. Therefore, concern over drug dependence should never be a reason to withhold adequate analgesia in patients suffering from acute post-operative or post-traumatic pain.

In summary, like all symptoms, acute pain usually reflects an underlying physiological disturbance, and should only be treated if the physician has an adequate understanding of the underlying pathology involved. Even if there is confidence in the diagnosis, the physician should periodically reevaluate the clinical process responsible for the pain. This will assure that the pain medications are not masking a disease entity that may be correctable with other therapeutic modalities. Such an exercise is especially prudent in those patients who do not obtain satisfactory relief with standard doses of analgesics.

CHRONIC PAIN

Chronic pain is that type of pain which is either persistent or episodic; the underlying cause is often not resolvable, is difficult to diagnose, or the pain may recur frequently. The effective management of chronic pain syndromes requires a great deal of therapeutic skill and constant reevaluation of the clinical situation. Although it is difficult to achieve completely, the ultimate treatment goal in the patient with chronic pain is to restore the individual's normal function within society. Therefore, physicians should strive to maintain treatment on an out-patient basis with therapeutic modalities that allow independence from the in-patient setting whenever possible.

One must remember that chronic pain is a multifactorial disorder and the disease process alone should not be the entire focus of the physician's endeavors. Assessment of other factors such as work-related and vocational pursuits and the possible need for utilization of vocational rehabilitation services as well as psychosocial aspects of chronic pain must be considered. Psychosocial aspects of chronic pain are among the most difficult problems to deal with in these patients. Issues such as home life, work, interpersonal relationships, financial disturbances, and other concurrent psychosocial problems (alcoholism, marital disputes, adult children of alcoholics, drug dependence, etc.) must be carefully assessed and addressed. To overlook these important factors in the treatment of chronic pain patients is to insure oneself a failure of treatment. More detailed information on the psychologic considerations in the management of chronic pain is available on pp. 86 - 93.

A National Institute of Health study showed that chronic pain was the most costly health problem in the United States, costing industries more than $50 billion per year. In another recent study, when the entire time lost secondary to back injury was taken into account, it was estimated that every working person in America would be able to take 75 days vacation per year if there was no time lost from back injury. Other studies have shown that headache is second only to urinary tract infections as the most frequent reason for doctor visits in the United States today.

To answer the question as to where do patients go when they have pain, the following have been reported: 55 percent of patients will go to a primary care physician or dentist, 25 percent to a chiropractor, 12 percent to a pharmacist, 5 percent to a podiatrist, and less than 3 percent to a pain management specialist. The subspecialty of pain management is relatively new and encompasses the disciplines of several medical specialties including anesthesiology, neurosurgery, neurology, clinical pharmacology, orthopedics, and rheumatology. Pain management centers generally treat a myriad of pain symptoms including cancer pain; reflex sympathetic dystrophy; back, head, and neck pain; facial pain; pain secondary to Herpes zoster (shingles); visceral pain; peripheral vascular disease; arthritis related pain; and pain with an unknown etiology. Pain management facilities can provide the advantage of a multidisciplinary approach to a patient's problem for the evaluation and treatment of the many problems that may co-exist in chronic pain patients.

Chronic pain can be subdivided on the basis of whether or not the underlying condition will affect the patient's life expectancy. The therapy for individuals whose life will be shortened by the condition, such as terminal cancer, will focus on the long-term use of opioids and adjuvant medications. In contrast, patients whose longevity will not be affected by the disease should be treated, for the most part, with non-opioid analgesics.

THERAPY OF CHRONIC BENIGN PAIN. The management of patients with chronic, but not life-shortening pain is a challenge which involves the appropriate use of non-opioid analgesics chosen in order to balance the pain relief obtained with the side effects that are associated with the compounds. It should be noted that the condition being treated is often progressive in nature, and that the patient must have the medication adjusted as the severity of the symptoms increases. Therapy is usually initiated with standard doses of aspirin, acetaminophen, or another NSAID as previously described for mild to moderate acute pain. Every effort must be made to maximize the analgesic benefit from these drugs. This usually requires at least one to two weeks of therapy before a particular therapeutic regimen is deemed unsuccessful. If this is the case, then the dose of the non-opioid agent used should be increased gradually; however, gastrointestinal intolerance usually limits the maximal NSAID dose in many patients. If this problem occurs, the concurrent administration of a gastrointestinal protective agent (such as sucralfate (CARAFATE), H_2-receptor blockers, oral antacids, or a specific protective agent such as misoprostol (CYTOTEC)) along with the NSAID may be of benefit, as described on pp. 66 - 67.

Other adjuvant medications may be crucial in the treatment of chronic benign pain in conjunction with the above recommendations. For example, muscle relaxants (see pp. 69 - 70) are highly effective in treating the muscle spasm component of pain. Side effects of these, such as sedation, are important to note when making a decision as to which agent to prescribe. Switching to a different muscle relaxant may be useful in reducing the annoying side effects while still allowing for the effective treatment of the muscle spasm. Tricyclic antidepressants (see p. 69) and other medications used in combination with NSAIDs are extremely beneficial. One must remember however, that adverse effects may be more common when using a combination drug regimen.

For those patients who have an inadequate response or unacceptable side effects to one NSAID, switching to an alternative NSAID may be helpful. The simultaneous administration of two NSAIDs have not been shown to be more efficacious than maximal doses of a single NSAID, however, at times, it does allow for minimizing an annoying side effect of one drug that prevents its sole use in a patient. The concurrent use of an NSAID and acetaminophen may produce additive analgesia since they apparently relieve pain by different mechanisms. Nevertheless, the long term administration of such combinations should be done with caution, since the risk of analgesic nephropathy from these mixtures is unknown. If the patient cannot tolerate any NSAID, then therapy with acetaminophen may have to suffice.

The regular use of opioid analgesics in benign pain syndromes is controversial. Some physicians would justify opioid use only in the short term management of acute, severe crises. Others advocate the continued use of opioids with a low dependence liability, such as agonist-antagonist agents, for patients who are resistant to, or suffer side effects from, non-opioid agents. Physicians who choose to use these types of opioids should be aware of the potential escalation by the patient to stronger types of medication during their treatment program. It is for these reasons that all efforts should be made not to utilize opioid treatment in these types of syndromes. The administration of strong opioids in chronic benign pain syndromes is to be avoided if at all possible, since the resulting problems of tolerance, physical dependence, and drug-seeking behavior are usually more life-disrupting than the pain process itself.

As stated above, some patients who are refractory to standard non-opioid drug regimens may obtain some additional relief by the coadministration of analgesic adjuvants (pp. 68 - 71). Others may obtain benefit from a neurosurgical or anesthetic procedure (pp. 73 - 80). All such refractory patients should be referred to a specialized pain management center where multidisciplinary management approaches are available. More detailed information on the therapy of three common benign pain syndromes (arthritis, low back pain, and trigeminal neuralgia) is provided on pp. 80 - 86.

CHRONIC PAIN IN CANCER PATIENTS. The management of chronic, cancer-related pain, is a common and often frustrating clinical situation. The World Health Organization listed the inadequate therapy of cancer-related pain as one of the most serious health problems in the world today. The goal of the physician should be to keep the patient relatively pain free, while allowing for as much normal functioning as possible. The adverse effects of treatment must, therefore, be balanced with the fear of recurring pain and its consequences, such as sleep disturbances, anorexia, anxiety, and depression. These conditions must often be treated separately with adjuvant medications as discussed on pp. 68 - 71.

Some patients with mild to moderate pain may be managed initially with acetaminophen, aspirin, or other NSAIDs. Well controlled studies in patients with moderate cancer pain have demonstrated that 650 mg of aspirin can be just as effective in relieving pain as a standard oral dose of codeine (30 to 60 mg). However, these non-opioid analgesics are often underutilized in the therapy of cancer-related pain. In many cancer patients, the non-opioids can have a significant opioid-sparing effect. NSAIDs can be particularly useful in the management of pain secondary to bony metastases, since they inhibit prostaglandin synthesis and release which has been shown to be involved in this situation. If NSAIDs are not used, pain secondary to bone metastases is extremely refractory to standard therapy.

Most patients with cancer-related pain will require opioids for pain relief at some point in the course of their illness. Initially, these patients can be managed effectively with the commonly used oral agents (codeine sulfate, oxycodone hydrochloride, a propoxyphene salt (DARVON or DARVON-N) or pentazocine hydrochloride (TALWIN NX)) in conjunction with a non-opioid compound. If the pain becomes refractory to these measures, the administration of a more potent opioid (e.g., morphine sulfate, hydromorphone hydrochloride (DILAUDID), and methadone hydrochloride (DOLOPHINE)) by the oral route should be initiated. Controlled release or sustained release preparations of morphine sulfate (e.g., MS CONTIN, ROXANOL) are very useful in avoiding the "peak and valley" effects that one may encounter with the shorter duration opioids. When using the sustained release preparations, dose adjustment may be made by allowing the patient to treat the "breakthrough" pain with an immediate release morphine sulfate preparation or another opioid analgesic.

The emphasis at this point should be on the *regular* administration of the oral opioids around-the-clock so that the fear of recurring pain is eliminated. The physician should be familiar with the duration of action of the medication prescribed so that drugs are administered at appropriate time intervals to maintain pain relief. In some instances, the patients should be awakened from sleep to take their medications. This approach should keep the pain at a tolerable level, and may actually decrease the 24-hour opioid requirement when compared to an "as needed" (prn) regimen. Prn dosage schedules most often result in "peak and valley" effects whereby the patient experiences significant adverse effects at the peak drug levels and inadequate pain relief at the valley blood concentrations prior to the next allowable dose. It is important to emphasize that sufficient medication must always be made available to the terminally ill patient.

Transdermal fentanyl (DURAGESIC) may prove to be as effective as oral or parenteral opioids for the treatment of chronic pain in cancer patients, although well-controlled studies which compare this preparation with other opioid analgesics are lacking. The use of the preparation is convenient, four dosage levels are available, and "peak and valley" blood levels are significantly reduced. However, achieving the proper dosage for the patient may be difficult and therapeutic blood concentration are usually not reached for 8 to 12 hours after the application of the first dose. In addition, when the dosage is increased it may require several days to reach a new steady-state equilibrium, and "breakthrough" pain may occur, necessitating the use of another opioid analgesic, oral or parenteral, during the titration period.

The choice of a potent oral opioid analgesic is arbitrary, and usually depends on the past experience of the patient and physician. When morphine sulfate, meperidine hydrochloride (DEMEROL), or hydromorphone hydrochloride (DILAUDID) are administered orally, they are approximately one-fourth to one-fifth as effective as when administered parenterally (see Table 3) and have a duration of action of about 4 hours. Nevertheless, all three agents, when administered orally, are very useful in the management of severe cancer-related pain, provided they are taken regularly in appropriate amounts. Typical starting doses are: 50 to 100 mg of meperidine hydrochloride (DEMEROL), 10 to 30 mg of morphine sulfate, or 2 to 4 mg of hydromorphone hydrochloride (DILAUDID) administered every 4 hours.

Caution should be exercised when giving meperidine hydrochloride to patients with any degree of renal impairment, since normeperidine, the major metabolite, will accumulate and possibly cause central nervous system toxicity such as seizures, tremors, and irritability. These complications have also occurred in patients with normal renal function receiving multiple meperidine doses. In addition, meperidine hydrochloride is the only opioid that has a direct effect on decreasing cardiac output and may lead to tachycardia. Therefore, this drug should be used with caution in patients with co-existing cardiac disease.

There was a lot of early enthusiasm about the use of oral methadone hydrochloride (DOLOPHINE) in the therapy of chronic cancer related pain because of its long plasma half-life. However, it has since been established that the duration of the analgesic effect of this drug is only about 6 hours, compared to its pharmacokinetic half-life of 24 hours. Therefore, to achieve adequate analgesia, methadone hydrochloride should probably be administered every 6 to 8 hours. Such a dosing schedule may cause delayed respiratory depression 3 to 4 days later, since the respiratory depressant effect of this compound is proportional to its plasma concentration, which will not reach a maximal steady-state level until at least 3 to 4 plasma half-lives. Because of this dichotomy between plasma and analgesic half-lives, careful dose titration with methadone hydrochloride is required in the initial dosing periods, in order to avoid drug accumulation to toxic levels; doses are usually titrated adequately by utilizing sedation as a guideline. Most commonly the dose of this drug may be reduced after the initial dosing period. Methadone continues to be one of the most effective agents in the management of these patients.

The dosages of all orally-administered potent opioids should be escalated gradually, in order to produce tolerable pain relief and minimal adverse effects. Once an acceptable regimen is achieved, many weeks may pass before the patient requires further dose escalation. However, most patients eventually have increased opioid requirements due to the development of tolerance or the progression of their disease. At this point, the physician should merely increase the dose of the drug to attain satisfactory analgesia without concern about the possibility of producing drug dependence in the patient. Some patients may eventually require large oral opioid doses, such as 20 mg of hydromorphone hydrochloride (DILAUDID) every 3 hours, or greater than 300 mg of morphine sulfate per day, in order to obtain adequate pain relief. These patients may still be managed on an outpatient basis for prolonged periods of time, provided opioid side effects are treated appropriately (see below). In those terminally-ill patients who can no longer take anything by mouth, administration of opioids via a rectal suppository, e.g., morphine sulfate, hydromorphone hydrochloride, or oxymorphone hydrochloride (see Table D, pp. 114 - 119), may delay the admission to the hospital for therapy with a parenteral opioid.

If the pain becomes so severe that it cannot be controlled with a regular schedule of potent oral or rectal opioids, or transdermal fentanyl, then the parenteral route must be employed. Any of the more potent agents can be used; however, agonist-antagonist agents should be avoided since they can precipitate opioid withdrawal in physically dependent patients. Hydromorphone hydrochloride (DILAUDID), administered intramuscularly, seems to have an advantage in this setting, since its high potency allows for a small injection volume. This is of particular concern for emaciated patients with low muscle mass. Finally, certain patients may require continuous intravenous opioids. Once again one should not forget the use of analgesic adjuvants, which allow for opioid sparing effects.

The use of epidural or intrathecal opioids can be of substantial benefit in the treatment of these patients allowing them an excellent quality of life and, in many cases, the ability to resume an almost normal life style. These catheters may be inserted percutaneously or implanted into the epidural space and tunneled subcutaneously to be connected to either an implanted reservoir with an external infusion device, or to an implanted refillable pump. These specialized pharmacologic approaches are discussed in more detail on pp. 72 - 73.

During an acute exacerbation of pain, while in the hospital, patient controlled analgesia (PCA) can be extremely helpful in controlling this problem in the patient to be afforded relief while diagnosis and treatment of the changing condition is in progress. It also allows the physician to better titrate back to oral opioid doses once the pain is under control with the PCA. PCA can be done with many parenteral opioids, but morphine sulfate is most commonly used. It may be used purely on demand, or with a small continuous dose and then allowing the patient the availability of a small (on demand) dose during movement to stretchers for transport, use of spirometry, etc. Most commonly PCA is employed under the direction of an anesthesiologist trained in its correct usage. PCA allows, once again, for avoidance of the "peak and valley" effects of prn medications.

MANAGEMENT OF CLINICAL PROBLEMS ASSOCIATED WITH OPIOID USE

The pharmacologic effects of opioid analgesics have been reviewed on pp. 17 - 36. This section will deal with ways to manage the undesirable effects of opioids clinically, so that the patient can receive maximum analgesia with the minimum of adverse reactions. In addition, special clinical situations will be considered in which particular opioid adverse reactions may be especially hazardous to the patient. The information in this section is outlined in Table 9.

RESPIRATORY DEPRESSION. The depressive effects of opioids on the respiratory drive are mediated by a direct action on the medullary respiratory center. Tolerance to this effect seems to develop at the same rate as tolerance to

TABLE 9. APPROACH TO CLINICAL PROBLEMS ASSOCIATED WITH OPIOID USE

PROBLEM	RECOMMENDED THERAPY
Respiratory Depression	Use a mixed agonist-antagonist opioid; check arterial blood gases and monitor vital signs frequently.
Constipation	Administer stool softeners and/or irritant cathartics (see Table P).
Sedation	Use small doses of the opioid at more frequent intervals; consider the use of daytime central nervous system stimulants.
Drug Allergy	Use parenteral antihistamines (see Table O), treat anaphylaxis, or switch to an opioid of a different chemical structure.
Nausea and Vomiting	Switch to another opioid; coadminister an antiemetic drug, e.g., prochlorperazine.
Tolerance	Switch to another opioid.
Physical Dependence	Reduce the dose of the opioid gradually; switch to either a less potent compound or methadone and reduce the dose slowly.

analgesia. Many studies have confirmed that all opioid agonists have comparable depressive effects on respiration when administered at equianalgesic parenteral doses. However, the opioid agonist-antagonists seem to be associated with less respiratory depression because of a "ceiling effect" on respiratory function.

For most patients, the effects on respiration are not clinically important. A 10 mg intramuscular dose of morphine sulfate will raise the pCO_2 by approximately 5 mm Hg, which is about equal to that which occurs during sleep. This response may be significant, however, for some elderly or debilitated patients, or those patients with obstructive airway disease or limited respiratory reserve of any etiology. In such patients, therapy with an agonist-antagonist agent may be preferable, and frequent monitoring of vital signs and mental status are recommended. Arterial blood gas measurements, if indicated, may be done at the time of peak drug effect. Any significant deterioration in respiratory function warrants immediate opioid reversal with titrated doses of naloxone hydrochloride (NARCAN). It should be remembered that with continued opioid use, drug accumulation, and therefore, increased respiratory depression will occur for a time period of up to 5 elimination half-lives (time to steady-state) of the particular opioid agent. Thus, continued close clinical monitoring should be undertaken during this time period. For these reasons, the initial use of oral opioid analgesics in outpatients with severe lung disease should be done only with careful consideration.

In some patients with increased intracranial pressure, such as those with acute head trauma or brain metastases, the CO_2 retention caused by opioid drugs may further elevate the cerebrospinal fluid pressure. Therefore, opioid analgesics should be used with extreme caution, and only when absolutely necessary, in these patients.

CONSTIPATION. The constipating effects of opioids on the bowel can sometimes be used to a clinical advantage, e.g., in the treatment of diarrhea; however, in general, constipation is a bothersome side effect. Particularly distressing is the fact that tolerance to the constipating effects of the opioids does not seem to occur as quickly as tolerance to analgesia. In order to avoid the more serious problems of ileus and fecal impaction, daily administration of both stool softeners and irritant cathartics are recommended (see Table P). Doses of these agents much higher than those commonly employed for routine bowel management may be necessary to offset the constipating effects of high doses of opioids. The use of opioids for the control of pain in conditions associated with toxic megacolon is absolutely contraindicated, since bowel perforation may ensue.

SEDATION. The sedative effects of opioid analgesics usually cannot be separated from their analgesic effects. An increase in dose will often cause a proportional increase in both analgesia and sedation. Sometimes these effects can be desirable, as is the case during the immediate postoperative period. However, in patients with subacute or chronic pain, such as burn or severe trauma victims, and in patients with terminal cancer, these effects are highly undesirable, since they can interfere with a patient's nutritional and rehabilitative care. Since the sedative effects of opioids are directly proportional to their plasma concentrations, one approach to this problem is to avoid high peak plasma levels by administering smaller doses at more frequent intervals. For example, if a person required 2 mg of hydromorphone hydrochloride (DILAUDID) parenterally every four hours, one could administer 1 mg every two hours during the daytime in an attempt to combat sedation. However, this technique may not work on every patient.

Again, patient controlled analgesia (PCA) may be extremely beneficial in reducing overall adverse effects by minimizing "peak and valley" effects and usually overall dosage. PCA may be continued at home if the patient has an indwelling intravenous or intraspinal (epidural or intrathecal) catheter. If sedation is interfering with a patient's progress, then some daytime analgesia may have to be sacrificed. Another approach is the concurrent use of stimulant drugs, e.g., dextroamphetamine or caffeine, during the day. Drugs that potentiate the sedative effects of opioids, such as benzodiazepines, phenothiazines, and antihistamines, may be reduced or stopped during the day.

DRUG ALLERGY. Minor allergic reactions to opioid analgesics are fairly common and are mediated, in part, by the propensity of these drugs to stimulate the release of histamine from tissue mast cells. Localized reactions, e.g., cutaneous rashes and pruritus, may be treated effectively with oral antihistamines and the appearance of these milder allergic states is not a reason for stopping the opioid, unless the problem becomes intolerable to the patient. The more severe systemic reactions, including anaphylaxis and bronchoconstriction, are usually the result of a hypersensitivity reaction to the particular opioid compound being used and are rarely seen. In this case, the condition should be treated immediately with intravenous epinephrine, antihistamines, and bronchodilators, and the use of the opioid analgesic should be terminated. Often, substituting a compound with a different chemical structure will solve the problem of drug hypersensitivity; for example, a patient who shows a hypersensitivity to codeine sulfate, a phenanthrene derivative, may be successfully switched to meperidine hydrochloride, a phenylpiperidine derivative.

NAUSEA AND VOMITING. These effects are mediated primarily by stimulation of the chemoreceptor trigger zone in the brain. The potential to produce nausea and vomiting varies with the individual agent in any given patient. Therefore, switching to an alternative opioid at an equianalgesic dose is a potential means of dealing with this problem. An alternative approach is to coadminister an antiemetic, such as prochlorperazine (COMPAZINE), promethazine (PHENERGAN), hydroxyzine (ATARAX, VISTARIL), or thiethylperazine (TORECAN), along with the opioid.

TOLERANCE. The time interval during which opioids can be administered before tolerance develops varies with the particular agent, the dose and frequency of administration, and the individual patient. In general, most patients receiving continuous high doses of opioids will become tolerant after about 10 days to two weeks of therapy. The earliest sign of tolerance is a complaint by the patient that the duration of effective analgesia has decreased or there exists ineffective analgesia. Traditionally, the dose of the opioid would then be escalated to provide adequate analgesia. However, there is now recent evidence that cross-tolerance is not complete for all opioids. Therefore, switching to another opioid at the first sign of tolerance is a reasonable first-step approach to this problem. For patients who are tolerant to large doses of a single opioid analgesic, changing to a different drug at a dose equal to one-half the equianalgesic dose (see Table 3, p. 23) is possible. Subsequent changes in dose are then based on the clinical response of the patient.

DEPENDENCE. Opioid dependence and subsequent withdrawal symptoms (pp. 25 and 26) are major complications which may occur during the use of these drugs. Opioid dependence, be it physical or psychological, is qualitatively and quantitatively different for certain groups of these analgesics. For example, dependence associated with butorphanol tartrate (STADOL), buprenorphine hydrochloride (BUPRENEX), dezocine (DALGAN), nalbuphine hydrochloride (NUBAIN), pentazocine lactate (TALWIN), and codeine is less than that of morphine. However, it is important to remember that, in many cases, patients can and will escalate their doses or change to a more potent opioid depending on the type of pain being treated. Most patients given an opioid for *acute pain* are usually able to discontinue the drug without difficulty; however, the dependency problem develops more commonly in patients who are being treated for *chronic pain*. When given potent opioids, patients will develop tolerance over a period of time and may experience dependence and withdrawal reactions within a few weeks of therapy. Once the physician is convinced that the patient has developed dependence toward the opioid, he/she must be very careful in his/her therapeutic approach toward the patient.

There are a number of methods available to assist the physician in managing this complicated problem. A few are: (1) slowly decreasing the dose of the drug; certain physicians utilize the guidelines of reducing the dose by 10 percent per week until the patient is asymptomatic, (2) switching to a less potent opioid, over a period of time, in conjunction with reducing the dose of the original agent; do not, however, suddenly stop the administration of the original drug, and (3) switching to a potent oral opioid such as methadone hydrochloride (DOLOPHINE) and then slowly lowering the dose of this drug (10 percent per week until the patient is asymptomatic). The advantages to methadone hydrochloride are that it is potent, effective orally and has a relatively long duration of action. In addition, patients who have been successfully converted to methadone, will have less chance of developing withdrawal symptoms if the dose is decreased slowly. This is mainly due to the slow clearance of the drug from the body, resulting in a slow tapering off of the effects. In comparison, morphine sulfate, which has a relative fast clearance, is more likely to cause withdrawal symptoms. It is important to remember not to administer a mixed agonist-antagonist opioid compound in dependent patients or a withdrawal reaction will be precipitated.

MANAGEMENT OF CLINICAL PROBLEMS ASSOCIATED WITH NSAID USE

The prolonged administration of most NSAIDs is generally considered to be safe and associated with an acceptable degree of side effects. However, in recent years, a number of clinical situations have been realized in which NSAID usage should be undertaken with caution. These special circumstances will be discussed briefly below and are summarized in Table 10.

TABLE 10. APPROACH TO CLINICAL PROBLEMS ASSOCIATED WITH NSAID USE

PROBLEM	RECOMMENDED THERAPY
Active peptic ulcer	Use a nonulcerogenic analgesic, e.g., acetaminophen, with or without an opioid analgesic.
History of peptic ulcer or gastrointestinal bleeding	Administer the NSAID with food, an antacid, sucralfate, or an H_2-receptor blocker (see Table Q); monitor clinical status closely.
Platelet abnormalities	Avoid NSAIDs.
Anticipated surgery	Discontinue NSAIDs (especially aspirin).
Concurrent warfarin therapy	Use ibuprofen, naproxen or tolmetin with caution; avoid phenylbutazone and salicylates.
Renal disease and low volume states	Do baseline urinalysis, electrolytes and creatinine; discontinue NSAID for weight gain, proteinuria or elevation in BUN, creatinine, or potassium.
Hypertension	Monitor blood pressure closely.
Geriatric patients	Watch closely for changes in mental status and discontinue NSAID for disorientation, irritability, depression, etc.

GASTROINTESTINAL DISEASE. Non-specific gastrointestinal symptoms of nausea, dyspepsia, epigastric pain, diarrhea, and abdominal cramps are among the most common side effects observed with NSAID use. In rarer instances, gastric or duodenal ulcers with gastrointestinal bleeding may develop. In general, most NSAIDs have less gastrointestinal side effects than equal anti-inflammatory doses of aspirin. However, to date, comparative clinical trials have not clearly delineated one particular NSAID as being the least toxic to the gastrointestinal tract.

Patients with a past history of peptic ulcer disease or gastrointestinal bleeding should only be given NSAIDs when frequent clinical monitoring is possible. One may consider the use of a less offensive agent, such as choline magnesium salicylate (TRILISATE), which may be better tolerated by these patients. If there is a history of gastrointestinal intolerance to one NSAID, then switching to an alternative compound may lessen the symptomatology. Administration of NSAIDs along with food, antacids (e.g., MAALOX, GELUSIL,

RIOPAN, etc.), sucralfate (CARAFATE) or H_2-receptor antagonists (cimetidine (TAGAMET), famotidine (PEPCID), nizatidine (AXID) and ranitidine (ZANTAC)), has been helpful for certain patients. A drug such as misoprostol (CYTOTEC) may also be beneficial in reducing the adverse gastrointestinal effects of NSAIDs when used concurrently (see Table Q). Since most NSAIDs are metabolized by the liver to inactive products, the concurrent administration of cimetidine (TAGAMET), by its inhibitory effect on drug metabolism, has the theoretical possibility of increasing NSAID plasma levels. Therefore, if an H_2-receptor blocker is desired in a patient receiving NSAIDs, one of the other drugs is probably a better choice.

In patients with active peptic ulcer disease and active rheumatoid arthritis, every effort should be made to treat the rheumatoid arthritis with a nonulcerogenic drug such as a gold compound. NSAIDs should be considered only if the benefits greatly outweigh the risks and if employed, they must be used only in stable patients receiving appropriate antiulcer therapy. Such patients should be closely supervised for the development of ulcer, gastrointestinal bleeding or perforation.

PLATELET ABNORMALITIES. All NSAIDs, by virtue of their effect on platelet eicosanoids, will inhibit platelet aggregation, and thus prolong the bleeding time. Aspirin acts irreversibly and will inhibit aggregation for the life of the platelet. Other NSAIDs have variable temporal platelet effects, which are sometimes dose-related. In general, all NSAIDs should be avoided in patients with qualitative or quantitative platelet abnormalities. Also, aspirin should be discontinued well in advance of any anticipated surgical procedure.

CONCURRENT WARFARIN THERAPY. All NSAIDs, by prolonging the bleeding time, may increase the risk of clinical bleeding in patients receiving oral anticoagulants. In addition, NSAIDs can cause gastric mucosal damage which may be potentially dangerous in an anticoagulated patient. Thus, all NSAIDs should be used with caution and only when absolutely necessary in patients treated with anticoagulant drugs. If one has to use an NSAID in a patient receiving warfarin (COUMARIN), the safest agents are probably ibuprofen (MOTRIN, etc.), naproxen (NAPROSYN), naproxen sodium (ANAPROX) and tolmetin sodium (TOLECTIN). Clinical studies have established that these drugs do not alter the hypoprothrombinemic response to warfarin. Ketorolac tromethamine (TORADOL) only slightly reduces the binding of warfarin to plasma proteins (99.3 percent as compared to the 99.5 percent control). Agents to be avoided are phenylbutazone and the salicylates; these compounds have definitely been shown to increase the risk of bleeding in patients receiving warfarin.

RENAL DISEASE AND LOW VOLUME STATES. Over the last several years, a full spectrum of renal complications including papillary necrosis, acute renal failure, the nephrotic syndrome, and interstitial nephritis have been recognized in patients receiving NSAIDs. Associated risk factors for the development of these syndromes include chronic renal insufficiency, renal vascular disease, and the low intravascular volume states associated with cirrhosis, congestive heart failure, the nephrotic syndrome, and diuretic therapy. Because of the prevalence of these conditions in the populations usually requiring NSAIDs, it is probably prudent to obtain a baseline urinalysis, and serum electrolytes and creatinine in all patients being started on chronic NSAID therapy. Frequent monitoring of clinical and laboratory indices should also be undertaken during the course of therapy. Weight gain, proteinuria, or an elevation in blood urea nitrogen (BUN), creatinine or potassium should alert the clinician to the possibility of NSAID-induced renal disease and warrant drug discontinuation.

HYPERTENSION. NSAIDs have been shown to block the effectiveness of some antihypertensive medications, especially diuretics. Therefore, to avoid uncontrolled hypertension, frequent blood pressure monitoring is advised in patients receiving concomitant therapy with antihypertensive agents and NSAIDs.

GERIATRIC PATIENTS. In general, elderly patients are more susceptible to adverse effects of NSAIDs than their younger counterparts. Geriatric patients seem to be particularly sensitive to changes in mental status associated with these drugs, such as disorientation, forgetfulness, irritability, depression, and paranoia. Clinicians should be especially aware of these symptoms, since drug discontinuation will result in a return to baseline mental status. One needs to remember that these problems may also be secondary to concomitant adjuvant medications (tricyclic antidepressants, antinauseants, skeletal muscle relaxants, antihistamines, etc).

SPECIALIZED PHARMACOLOGIC APPROACHES TO PAIN

Despite the potent analgesic properties of both the opioids and NSAIDs, there exists, unfortunately, a large number of individuals who still experience significant amounts of pain even with optimal use of these agents. The reasons for these failures are many, but are usually related to drug tolerance or side effects. This section describes innovative pharmacologic methods of pain therapy which may be of some benefit to those patients who fail to response to more traditional measures.

ANALGESIC ADJUVANTS

Adjuvants to pain therapy offer a valuable addition to the treatment modalities available to the physician. This group of compounds can be divided into a number of different pharmacologic categories including central nervous system stimulants, antidepressants, spasmolytic agents, skeletal muscle relaxants, antipsychotics, antihistamines, anxiolytics, anticonvulsants, and antiarrhythmic agents. The mechanism of analgesic action of these drugs is frequently conjectural, and critical proof of analgesic efficacy is often inconclusive. However, there are clinical situations where adjuvant therapy may provide substantial analgesic benefit to the patient. It is interesting that as our understanding of pain transmission mechanisms improves, some of the empirical observations of adjuvant drug therapy have acquired scientific validity. Table N lists the most frequently used analgesic adjuvant medications based on current clinical studies.

STIMULANTS AND ANTIDEPRESSANTS. The use of central nervous system stimulants and antidepressant drugs, in the treatment of various pain syndromes, has not been widely accepted; this appears to be due to the physician's fear of drug dependence and potential central nervous system stimulatory side effects. However, there are certain specific situations, where these drugs have been found to be extremely effective, e.g., when there is excessive sedation induced by the opioid analgesic or when there is a strong depressant component to the illness.

Of all of the central nervous system stimulants, caffeine and dextroamphetamine are the most popular. By the oral route, dextroamphetamine sulfate (DEXEDRINE), at a dose of 5 to 10 mg in the morning, is especially useful in combatting the daytime sedation induced by opioid analgesics. The combination of morphine sulfate (12 mg, IM) and dextroamphetamine sulfate (10 mg, IM), has been found to be twice as effective for analgesia as morphine sulfate alone. Caffeine, a constituent of both over-the-counter and prescription medications, is an effective analgesic adjuvant at doses of at least 65 mg. In combination with various non-opioid analgesics, such as aspirin or acetaminophen, caffeine has been demonstrated to increase their analgesic activity.

Tricyclic antidepressants, such as amitriptyline (ELAVIL, ENDEP), imipramine (TOFRANIL), and nortriptyline (AVENTYL), are commonly used adjuvants in the treatment of depression associated with chronic pain. Some investigations have demonstrated that the tricyclic antidepressants have a potent analgesic activity of their own, but also potentiate other analgesics as well. The mechanism appears to be related to three major actions: (1) a serotonergic sparing action, (2) alteration in the number of opioid receptors available for drug binding, and (3) increasing the efficacy of the opioid agonist binding to opioid receptors. These antidepressants appear to be beneficial in the treatment of chronic pain; the clinical efficacy of these compounds, used either alone or in combination therapy, in the treatment of post-herpetic neuralgia, migraine, and chronic tension headaches, has been substantiated.

SKELETAL MUSCLE RELAXANTS. The skeletal muscle relaxants can be divided into two major categories, (1) the spasmolytic agents, and (2) the centrally-acting skeletal muscle relaxants. The primary spasmolytic agents are diazepam (VALIUM) and baclofen (LIORESAL), which act in the spinal cord, and dantrolene sodium (DANTRIUM), which acts directly on skeletal muscle. These drugs are all effective in reducing muscle spasticity, which leads to a reduction in pain. The choice of the agent to be used depends upon the condition being treated, associated illnesses, and potential drug interactions.

The centrally-acting skeletal muscle relaxants include carisoprodol (SOMA), chlorphenesin carbamate (MAOLATE), chlorzoxazone (PARAFLEX, PARAFON FORTE DSC), cyclobenzaprine hydrochloride (FLEXERIL), methocarbamol (ROBAXIN) and orphenadrine citrate (NORFLEX). The basic mechanism of these drugs for the relief of pain is related to their ability to decrease muscular spasms. The use of these compounds is only part of an entire therapeutic regimen which may include physical therapy and orthopedic procedures. In combination with certain other drugs, such as aspirin, acetaminophen, and caffeine, some centrally-acting skeletal muscle relaxants are promoted as having an increased effect in situations where there is considerable tissue damage, pain, and edema.

ANTIPSYCHOTIC AND ANTIANXIETY AGENTS. Antipsychotic drugs and antianxiety agents (anxiolytics) are used as adjuvants for the treatment of pain due to their ability to alter the behavioral status of the pain patient. Obviously, in certain chronic situations, where psychosis or anxiety is a prime constituent of the clinical picture, these drugs become very useful. Drugs such as fluphenazine (PROLIXIN) and haloperidol (HALDOL) are examples of the antipsychotics. Of the anxiolytic group of drugs, the benzodiazepines, e.g., alprazolam (XANAX), appears to be the most useful. It still remains unclear as to whether any of these drugs have intrinsic analgesic activity, if they potentiate other analgesics, or if they change the patient's perception of pain. Their main value is in the treatment of other symptoms, such as anxiety, often associated with the pain patient. Buspirone hydrochloride (BUSPAR), a non-benzodiazepine anxiolytic drug, may be extremely useful as an adjuvant agent. It has few side effects, is not habit-forming, and is generally well tolerated; the major drawback of this drug is its slow onset of clinical effectiveness (1 to 6 weeks), which may deleteriously affect patient compliance.

ANTIHISTAMINES. The major antihistamine which has been used as an adjuvant in the therapy of pain is hydroxyzine (ATARAX, VISTARIL). It is the only antihistamine proven to have intrinsic analgesic activity of its own; it also potentiates the effects of analgesics, especially opioids. Generally, the drug is given in doses of 50 to 100 mg, orally or intramuscularly, along with an opioid analgesic. Some clinicians feel that the sedative effect of the antihistamine enhances the sedative activity of the opioid and is the major benefit of this combination. Oral hydroxyzine alone is also useful as a non-addicting, anxiolytic agent in the management of chronic pain syndromes.

ANTICONVULSANTS. The anticonvulsant drugs have been demonstrated to be effective in certain types of neurological pain, including phantom limb pain, the thalamic syndrome, or lightning tabetic pain. The drugs most often prescribed include carbamazepine (TEGRETOL) and phenytoin sodium (DILANTIN). Valproic acid (DEPAKENE) or its sodium salt, i.e., divalproex sodium (DEPAKOTE), are anticonvulsants that have demonstrated satisfactory analgesic activity; the myriad of adverse effects, however, lessen their utility for this purpose. When any of the anticonvulsant drugs are used, patients must have baseline blood studies performed and be monitored at regular intervals. In addition, because of the number of side effects and potential drug interactions, the physician should be thoroughly familiar with the pharmacological properties of these agents prior to their use.

ANTIARRHYTHMICS. Some antiarrhythmic agents have been used in the treatment of chronic pain. For example, bretylium tosylate (BRETYLOL) has been used in conjunction with an intravenous regional block for the therapy of reflex sympathetic dystrophy of the upper or lower extremities. It is used in a dose of approximately 1 mg/kg added to an appropriate volume of preservative-free 0.5% lidocaine. Mexiletine hydrochloride (MEXITIL) has shown some promising effectiveness in the treatment of chronic pain states, especially post-herpetic neuralgia refractory to other medications and repetitive sympathetic blockade, as well as in some other neuropathic states. It is used orally as 100 mg tid initially and the dose is increased to a point of efficacy up to 600 mg tid. Generally, it may be necessary to titrate the dose to the point of mild toxicity (e.g., tremors, irritability) and then decrease the dose one step and maintain the chronic dosage there. Once again there have been no overall controlled studies in the use of these agents and it is strongly recommended that these drugs be utilized only by physicians familiar with them.

CONTINUOUS INTRAVENOUS OPIOIDS

The continuous intravenous administration of opioid analgesics has become popular in recent years. This method is most useful for those terminally ill cancer patients who cannot take oral medications or who are not candidates for implantable intraspinal devices. It should be emphasized however, that the chronic intravenous administration of opioids should be reserved for completely uncontrolled pain as a "last resort." The use of newer opioid agents, as well as sustained release preparations, along with the adjuvant medications and implantable intraspinal devices generally makes the use of continuous intravenous opioids unnecessary. Morphine sulfate and meperidine hydrochloride (DEMEROL) are the two agents most commonly used. In non-tolerant patients of average weight with acute pain, the usual doses of morphine sulfate and meperidine hydrochloride are 3 mg/hr and 20 mg/hr, respectively. Some patients with severe acute pain may require higher doses. However, increasing the infusion rate more than once a day should be done with extreme caution, since the new peak opioid plasma level will not be attained until 12 to 24 hours (time to steady-state) after a rate change. Thus, with any adjustment in dose, there is always the chance of causing delayed respiratory depression 12 to 24 hours later. Frequent assessment of vital signs is mandatory during this period, and naloxone should be available for the immediate reversal of opioid-induced toxicity. Patients with chronic cancer-related pain can become rapidly tolerant, and require hourly analgesic doses substantially higher than those administered for acute pain.

For the therapy of postoperative pain, some hospitals are using patient-controlled intravenous injection systems (or patient-controlled analgesia, PCA), an approach which allows the patient to titrate the dose of the analgesic according to his or her individual needs. These systems consist of either variable rate intravenous infusions or self-triggered intravenous bolus injections. A dose range of the opioid is predetermined by the physician, and safety devices are incorporated into the equipment which prevent accidental overdosage. Thus, the patients are limited as to the amount of drug which can be self-administered. Many studies have demonstrated that PCA in the early postoperative period is safe and provides superior analgesia compared to intermittent intramuscular injections.

EPIDURAL AND INTRATHECAL OPIOIDS

By means of catheters introduced into the epidural and intrathecal spaces, clinicians can now control pain by infusing opioid analgesics into selected areas of the spinal cord. The agents appear to act by binding to specific opioid receptors in the spinal cord. The method is very efficacious in the therapy of postoperative, obstetrical and chronic cancer pain, and the reports with this approach are encouraging. A rare, but serious, adverse effect which may occur with the use of intraspinal opioids is respiratory depression. Respiratory depression is produced by rostral spread of the opioid into the brain. The respiratory depression is usually delayed, and can occur up to 12 hours after the dose. Its onset is insidious and is more common in geriatric patients and in patients with pulmonary disease, especially in those with chronic obstructive pulmonary disease (COPD). Its usual precedent sign is increasing sedation or changes in cerebration (confusion). The respiratory depression is commonly associated with the concomitant use of parenteral opioids. Although the use of concomitant parenteral opioids is occasionally necessary in the management of cancer patients, this should be handled by physicians specifically trained in the subspecialty of pain management. To date, there are no reports of clinically significant respiratory depression in chronic pain patients. Less serious side effects of intraspinal opioid administration include nausea, pruritus and urinary retention. All of these adverse effects can be reversed by the use of antihistamines, antinauseants or naloxone.

Morphine sulfate, meperidine hydrochloride (DEMEROL), fentanyl citrate (SUBLIMAZE), hydromorphone hydrochloride (DILAUDID), methadone hydrochloride (DOLOPHINE) and β-endorphin are all effective analgesics by both the epidural and intrathecal routes. Morphine sulfate is the agent most commonly used, because it seems to produce the longest duration of analgesia (12 to 36 hours). For acute pain, the dose of morphine sulfate varies from 0.2 to 2 mg (by intrathecal administration) and 2 to 10 mg (by the epidural route).

The continuous use of epidural fentanyl was first popularized in 1982. It is mixed in preservative-free normal saline at a concentration of 10 μg/mL. The usual dose is 1 μg/kg per hour (0.1 mL/kg per hour). The dose is titrated up or down by efficacy versus side effects and is related to the point of placement of the epidural catheter. Fentanyl is a very lipid soluble agent, unlike morphine sulfate which is very water soluble. This accounts for the significant decrease in overall adverse effects with fentanyl and its segmental effect. The closer the catheter is to the dermatomal distribution of pain, generally the less total dose necessary to provide adequate pain relief. Patients on epidural opioids should be monitored for changes in cerebral or respiratory status.

For patients with chronic cancer-related pain, permanent catheters can be implanted in the subarachnoid and epidural spaces and connected to reservoirs or perfusion pumps. These devices allow for continuous outpatient analgesic therapy with spinal opioids. This method was originally restricted to patients with limited life expectancy, but secondary to advances in implantable technology and its overall excellent results; it is now considered useful in the earlier phases of cancer pain management, especially to avoid the problems associated with "polypharmacy." Intraspinal opioids have no effect on the progression of the disease and only serve to improve the quality of life. In many cases, the change in quality of life is impressive — almost comatose patients on intravenous opioids have been rendered pain free and able to resume the performance of activities of daily living. Many patients have even been able to return to work. Intraspinal opioids are considered by pain management specialists to be the technique of choice before any thought of parenteral opioids or neurolytic/neuroablative procedures.

NEUROSURGICAL APPROACHES TO PAIN

Neurosurgical techniques in the management of pain are based on current neuroanatomic and neurophysiologic knowledge of pain transmission and perception and the advances in these methods have paralleled the progression of our understanding of pain. Today, most procedures are performed percutaneously, without the need for general anesthesia and its associated risks. There are three basic neurosurgical approaches in the treatment of pain: (1) interruption of pain pathways which process pain from the periphery to the higher brain centers (Table 11), (2) stimulation of inhibitory modulating pathways which inhibit pain transmission (Table 12), and (3) the introduction of opioid analgesics via a catheter into the area surrounding the spinal cord. This procedure, which may include the

TABLE 11. NEUROSURGICAL PROCEDURES EMPLOYED TO INTERRUPT PAIN TRANSMISSION

LOCATION	DESTRUCTIVE TECHNIQUE	DESCRIPTION
Peripheral Nerve	Peripheral Neurotomy	Transection of peripheral nerve.
Posterior Root	Rhizotomy (Radicotomy)	Transection of the dorsal root between the spinal cord and the spinal ganglion. Percutaneous controlled thermocoagulation of the dorsal roots is also performed. This allows some selectivity for analgesia without complete anesthesia. This principle is based on the selective elimination of the nonmyelinated or lightly myelinated pain conducting fibers (A-delta and C fibers) which are more sensitive to heat than the more myelinated fibers involved in other sensory modalities.
Spinal Cord	Cordotomy	Destruction of the ascending tract systems in the anterolateral part of the spinal cord. Bilateral cordotomy may be performed, but unlike unilateral cordotomy, the side effects are frequent and potentially serious.
	Myelotomy	Interruption of the ventral commissure which contains the decussating spinothalamic tract fibers.
	Dorsal Root Entry Zone Lesion	Lesions are made in the dorsal root entry zone with a laser or radiofrequency probe.
Brain Stem	Medullary Tractotomy	Disruption of the trigeminal nerve tract in the medulla oblongata for pain in the face or pharynx.
	Mesencephalotomy	Destruction of the mesencephalic portion of the spinothalamic tract.
Thalamus	Thalamotomy	Selective ablation of specific thalamic nuclei considered part of the nonspecific pain pathway.
Pituitary	Hypophysectomy	Elimination of the hypophysis can reduce pain, especially when pain is associated with hormone dependent carcinoma. Numerous operative approaches are available for ablation of the pituitary, including transcranial, transsphenoidal, cryosurgical, radioactive implantation, and (most recently) transsphenoidal injection of alcohol.

TABLE 12. NEUROSURGICAL PROCEDURES EMPLOYED TO STIMULATE ANALGESIA

LOCATION	STIMULATORY TECHNIQUE	DESCRIPTION
Peripheral	Transcutaneous Electrical Nerve Stimulation (TENS)	Electrical devices placed on the skin over the affected area or at specific acupuncture points, stimulate nerve fibers.
Spinal Cord	Dorsal Column Stimulation	Electrodes are implanted percutaneously into the dorsal epidural space.
	Epidural Stimulation	An open surgical procedure with electrodes sewn onto the dura mater.
Intracerebral	Periaqueductal Grey Stimulation	Electrical stimulation of the periventricular and periaqueductal grey matter.
	Thalamic Simulation	Electrodes are implanted in various thalamic sensory nuclei.

implantation of a subcutaneous reservoir to allow continuous infusion of opioids, was discussed above under: EPIDURAL AND INTRATHECAL OPIOIDS.

The neurosurgical approach for the relief of pain is specifically designed as a tertiary therapeutic measure. Individuals suffering from chronic or acute pain should be treated in a more conservative manner before neurosurgery is undertaken. While these techniques will result in pain relief in some patients, generally neuroablative procedures have proven to be unsatisfactory secondary to inadequate pain relief, recurrence of pain at a later date, or unacceptable side effects. Failures of specific procedures have demonstrated our inadequate understanding of pain processing and transmission.

ANESTHETIC MEASURES FOR THE TREATMENT OF PAIN

Anesthetic approaches provide an alternative treatment modality for the pain patient and are primarily used for pain control in chronic disease states. These procedures are based on either (a) blockade of conduction of nerve impulses transmitting the noxious stimulus by the use of local anesthetics, or (b) destruction of participating nerve fibers by infiltration of neurolytic agents. Many of the techniques utilized for anesthetic relief of pain are accompanied by potentially serious side effects and should be employed by a highly trained, skilled anesthesiologist. The procedures performed can be divided into specific categories: (1) myofascial trigger point injection, (2) peripheral nerve block, (3) autonomic plexi block, (4) inhalation analgesia, (5) neurolytic blockade, (6) implantation of intraspinal opioid devices, and (7) implantation of spinal cord stimulation devices.

Local anesthetic agents, such as lidocaine hydrochloride (XYLOCAINE HCL) or bupivacaine hydrochloride (MARCAINE HCL), administered in sufficient concentration, will reduce or block the conduction of nerve impulses. This neuronal inhibition is a function of numerous factors including anesthetic potency, anesthetic concentration, myelin sheath size, and nerve fiber diameter. There is selective inhibition of the pain fibers, which are thinly myelinated and of a small diameter when compared to the motor and proprioceptive fibers. Selective blockade can be attained by the utilization of a less concentrated anesthetic solution or a lower dose. This selectivity is a general principle and variations can lead to unexpected adverse effects, e.g., motor weakness and autonomic dysfunction. The duration of analgesia is also a function of multiple factors including drug biotransformation, molecular structure of the local anesthetic, tissue vascularity, and receptor affinity. Epinephrine may be added to the local anesthetic solution to prolong the effective interval of anesthetic blockade; the addition of this potent vasoconstrictor causes a reduction in local blood flow and subsequently decreases the absorption of the local anesthetic from the injection site. However, epinephrine can cause significant side effects when sufficient quantities are absorbed systemically, e.g., tachycardia, hypertension, and panic attacks. Long acting local anesthetic agents, such as bupivacaine hydrochloride or etidocaine hydrochloride (DURANEST HCL), have been more popular than the combination of epinephrine and the local anesthetic.

Neurolytic agents are used to cause irreversible damage to neurological tissue. Two agents commonly utilized for neurolysis are absolute ethanol (ethyl alcohol) and phenol. Absolute ethanol acts instantaneously and disrupts all of the neural elements regardless of the myelin sheath thickness. It causes a significant perineural inflammatory response which can cause pain and scarring. Alcohol utilization in the peripheral nervous system is generally confined to specific indications, e.g., sensory nerves or post-amputation stump pain. The exception is in the therapy of refractory spasticity such as that found in spastic paraplegia. Peripheral nerves may be neurolysed by either ethanol or phenol, thus decreasing the amount of spasms and pain. Ethanol is used in a concentration of 50 to 100 percent.

Intrathecal injections of alcohol must be performed by skilled anesthesiologists and the techniques used emphasize proper positioning of the patient. Absolute alcohol is hypobaric when compared to cerebrospinal fluid; this causes alcohol injected into the subarachnoid space to move rapidly to the uppermost portion of the spinal canal. Therefore, the patient must be positioned so that the intrathecal injection of alcohol will diffuse to the sensory target structures, avoiding the motor or other sensory modalities. Because of the nonspecific effects of alcohol and potential adverse neuronal effects, intrathecal alcohol injections are designed for specific cases.

Phenol is a less potent neurolytic agent; it is used in a concentration of 5 to 10 percent. Initially, a latent period occurs which produces a reversible local anesthetic effect. At the end of this latent period, irreversible neurolysis occurs. Phenol also exhibits specificity in the destruction of nerve fibers; when used in proper concentrations it can interrupt thin myelinated fibers (sympathetic or sensory fibers) while sparing fibers enveloped in thick myelin (motor fibers). This allows selectivity for pain fibers while avoiding motor and proprioceptive elements. Phenol can be prepared with distilled water or normal saline for selective peripheral neurolysis or with glycerol, generally for intrathecal administration. When combined with glycerol, the preparation is hyperbaric when compared to cerebrospinal fluid. Therefore, in contrast to absolute alcohol, the target neural tissue must be in the dependent part of the spinal fluid compartment. Again, careful positioning of the patient is critical for success.

Epiduralysis can also be performed by the placement of a special catheter in the epidural space via the caudal approach. Administration of 10 percent hypertonic saline and methylprednisolone is done to lyse adhesions related to epidural fibrosis associated with nerve root compression and provide mild, short-term reversible sensory neurolysis.

MYOFASCIAL TRIGGER POINT INJECTION. This anesthetic procedure is common to clinical practice and is often performed outside the hospital setting. A local anesthetic such as bupivacaine hydrochloride (MARCAINE HCL) is infiltrated into the trigger point, where touch or pressure will elicit pain; pain originating from a localized trigger point is reproducible and distributed in a nondermatomal pattern. The trigger point may be directly related to the malignant process, trauma or as a sequelae to treatment modalities. Symptoms may be vague, generally radiating and may be associated with nondescriptive neurological symptoms such as numbness or paresthesias. It may also progress to autonomic dysfunction with resultant development of reflex sympathetic dystrophy. This type of pain responds poorly to opioid and non-opioid analgesic medications alone, but readily responds to local anesthetic infiltration, with analgesia lasting for more than several hours. It should be treated with a combination of medications, physical therapy, and reconditioning exercises, modality usage, relaxation training, and neural blockade. Myofascial pain is part of a pain syndrome and is common to patients suffering terminal, rheumatologic and post-traumatic (e.g., whiplash) diseases. These patients often have muscular imbalances secondary to therapeutic interventions, postural changes, malnutrition, and prolonged bed rest. All of these factors are abnormal stressors on the musculoskeletal system and can lead to myofascial pain.

PERIPHERAL NERVE BLOCKS. Chronic pain syndromes usually do not affect a single nerve or one spinal dermatomal distribution; however, there are specific circumstances when this may occur. For example, (1) spinal root pain in reflex sympathetic dystrophy (RSD) or post-laminectomy adhesions, and (2) peripheral nerve involvement in carpal tunnel syndrome or post-herpetic neuralgia, or post-traumatic neuropathy. Also, carcinoma may impinge on a specific nerve causing pain in a dermatomal distribution. In these circumstances, a peripheral nerve block would be a viable treatment choice for pain relief. This nerve block may be employed as a therapeutic modality or as a diagnostic procedure to identity the dermatomal areas involved for subsequent neurolysis. Often, the anesthetic to be administered (such as bupivacaine hydrochloride) is combined with a corticosteroid (e.g., methylprednisolone) to provide an anti-inflammatory component to the treatment. The pain relief is usually instantaneous and the duration of action may be prolonged or permanent. Recurrent pain can be treated with repeated injections of the local anesthetic, neurolysis with alcohol or phenol, or interruption of the nerve by a cryogenic or surgical technique.

Remember, cancer patients may exhibit signs and symptoms of other pain syndromes as well as myofascial pain syndrome and RSD. In addition, abrupt changes in symptomatology should alert the physician that coexisting disease must be ruled out. For example, a patient with acute onset of paresthesias or back, neck or extremity pain may have a herniated disc or a symptomatic metastasis.

Lumbar or caudal epidurals may be beneficial in many disease states. These would include (1) diseases that have failed conservative or usual medical therapy (e.g., diabetic neuropathy or certain headache states), (2) as therapy prior to surgical intervention (e.g., herniated disc), (3) therapy after surgical intervention has failed (e.g., failed back surgery syndrome/post laminectomy pain or pain secondary to rectal sigmoid cancer), or (4) disease states in which epidural sympathetic blockade is the initial therapy of choice (post-herpetic neuralgia or central herniated disc).

AUTONOMIC PLEXI BLOCK. Various autonomic plexi may be involved in the perpetuation of chronic pain. One of the most widely performed autonomic blocks is the celiac plexus block for midabdominal pain associated with pancreatic carcinoma. The three principal targets utilized to interrupt the regional sympathetic nerve supply are: (1) cervico-thoracic sympathetic block (stellate ganglion), (2) celiac-splanchnic block (celiac plexus), and (3) lumbar paravertebral sympathetic block. Sympathetic blocks are employed to alter pain perception mainly through their peripheral vasomotor effects. Following autonomic blockade and subsequent pain relief, a continued series of sympathetic blockades are quite successful in curing most disease states involving RSD. Sympathetic blocks must be performed as part of an overall treatment program including medications (NSAID, calcium channel blockers such as nifedipine (PROCARDIA), tricyclic antidepressants), physical therapy including rehabilitation, and modality usage such as transcutaneous electrical nerve stimulation (TENS), psychosocial interaction with stress management and dermal biofeedback. To expect one modality alone to be effective in treating such a complex disease syndrome as reflex sympathetic dystrophy (RSD) is foolhardy at best. Continuous sympathetic blockade via placement of an indwelling brachial plexus, epidural, or lumbar sympathetic catheter is also also very effective in treating cases of RSD or cases involving the need for considerable manipulation or mobilization of joints. In rare instances (usually long-standing cases that have persisted unreferred prior to therapy), neurolysis, either chemically or surgically, may be employed. The overall highest success rate for surgical sympathectomy reported is 86 percent. Chemical neurolysis generally provides a higher probability of success, especially when performed with radiologic or CT guidance. Both techniques carry different but significant risks and the outcome is most dependent on the performer's experience and technique.

The early referral of RSD for evaluation treatment is essential for a successful outcome. Unfortunately, since RSD most commonly results from quite minor injuries (sprains, casting, etc.) as well as from serious trauma (crush injuries, post myocardial infarction, post cerebrovascular accidents, etc.), significant time may elapse prior to referral for diagnosis or treatment. In addition, since diagnostic studies may be negative and pain may be the most significant presenting finding, these patients are often doomed to the mistake of a psychiatric diagnosis instead of the correct diagnosis. Needless to say, evaluation and treatment should be by a qualified pain management specialist.

INHALATION ANALGESIA. Certain inhalation general anesthetics have potent analgesic effects and are useful in certain clinical situations. Nitrous oxide is an effective analgesic agent when administered by inhalation. A mixture of 25 percent nitrous oxide with 75 percent oxygen gives substantial pain relief with minor disturbance in consciousness.

SPINAL CORD STIMULATION. The placement of an electrode in the epidural space to provide continuous or cyclic stimulation can be very effective in treating chronic pain states. There are three specific indications for spinal cord stimulation: (1) causalgia/resistant RSD, (2) failed back surgery syndrome with light pain, and (3) vasospastic or peripheral vascular disease. Systems can be totally implanted utilizing pacemaker-type technology or partially implanted using an external transmitter. Spinal cord stimulation can provide dramatic relief of the pain associated with these chronic debilitating conditions and may be placed by a neurosurgeon or by an anesthesiologist trained in the subspecialty of pain management.

THERAPY OF REPRESENTATIVE BENIGN PAIN SYNDROMES

ARTHRITIS

Arthritis is an inflammatory process within a joint space that may be a primary disease process or a component of many medical syndromes. The most common types of arthritis encountered by the physician are osteoarthritis and rheumatoid arthritis. Osteoarthritis is also called degenerative joint disease, because its pathogenesis is linked to age-related destruction of articular cartilage. Rheumatoid arthritis is a multisystem disorder with an arthritic component, that is characterized by a severely inflamed joint lining with resultant destruction of bone and cartilage. A brief pharmacologic approach to alleviating the pain associated with these two disorders is described below.

OSTEOARTHRITIS. The therapy of osteoarthritis should include a complete program designed to relieve pain and minimize disability and progression of the disease process. Non-pharmacologic measures should include weight reduction to ideal weight and carefully selected exercise to maintain joint function. Since osteoarthritis often has an inflammatory component, NSAIDs are probably preferable to acetaminophen for pain relief in those patients that can tolerate them. Aspirin is usually the first-line drug because of its low cost. However, in patients who prefer to take medication less often, any of the longer-acting NSAIDs, e.g., diflunisal (DOLOBID), nabumetone (RELAFEN), naproxen (NAPROSYN), oxaprozin (DAYPRO), or piroxicam (FELDENE), can be used. The minimal dose that produces effective analgesia should be employed. Many patients will only require aspirin or other NSAIDs on an "as needed basis". In general, every effort should be made to avoid using opioid analgesics. Systemic corticosteroids should also be avoided. Occasional intra-articular injections of insoluble steroids such as methylprednisolone acetate suspension (DEPO-MEDROL) with a local anesthetic, such as lidocaine, can be justified in certain patients with severe, intermittent, acute inflammatory flares.

RHEUMATOID ARTHRITIS. The primary goals of rheumatoid arthritis therapy are the elimination of pain and inflammation, maintenance of joint mobility, and prevention of deformity. Initial treatment usually consists of an anti-inflammatory dose of a salicylate designed to achieve a therapeutic salicylate level of 20 to 25 mg/dL. This usually requires administering at least 12 aspirin tablets daily (3 with each meal and 3 at bedtime). However, some patients may require up to 20 aspirin tablets per day to achieve adequate relief. In settings where the measurement of serum salicylate levels is not readily available, the aspirin dose is usually titrated upward until the patient develops gastrointestinal side effects or tinnitus. If prolonged administration of large doses of plain aspirin leads to mild gastrointestinal intolerance (nausea, dyspepsia, diarrhea) switching to other salicylate preparations, (e.g., choline magnesium salicylate (TRILISATE), or salsalate (DISALCID)), or enteric coated preparations of aspirin (e.g., ECOTRIN) may cause fewer gastrointestinal side effects.

If patients prefer to take medications less often, therapy can be initiated with any of the longer-acting non-pyrazolon NSAIDs (Table H, pp. 124 - 134). If there is an inadequate response or adverse effects to one NSAID, then sometimes switching the patient to an alternative NSAID can be of benefit. Many patients with rheumatoid arthritis will require extended and even life-long therapy with NSAIDs. These patients are much more susceptible to adverse effects than those patients taking short courses of these drugs for acute pain. Thus the physician should constantly monitor appropriate clinical and laboratory parameters in these patients. A discussion of adverse effects of the NSAIDs and their management is provided on pp. 65 - 68. In the future, routine measurement of serum NSAID levels may be helpful in titrating NSAID dosages in individual patients so as to maximize analgesia and minimize adverse effects. It should be remembered that NSAIDs only treat the inflammatory symptoms of rheumatoid arthritis; there is no convincing evidence that these drugs alter the course of the disease process. Warm water exercise and/or physical therapy such as that provided by arthritis patient services is very beneficial in increasing the range of motion and decreasing the pain of the inflamed joints. Its use may make a resistant case of rheumatoid or osteoarthritis much more amenable to treatment.

Patients with rapidly progressive and destructive disease not responsive to adequate courses of NSAIDs should be treated with disease-modifying drugs in an attempt to diminish joint destruction; auranofin (RIDAURA), aurothioglucose (SOLGANAL), hydroxychloroquine sulfate (PLAQUENIL SULFATE), and methotrexate are agents in this category. Since all of these compounds have potentially serious toxicities, including dermatitis, the nephrotic syndrome, retinopathy, bone marrow suppression, and immunosuppression, they should only be administered by physicians experienced with their use.

LOW BACK PAIN

Low back pain affects approximately 80 percent of all individuals at some time during their lives. Many studies claim low back pain to be the leading cause of chronic disability and industrial absenteeism. All primary care physicians should be competent in the initial evaluation of the painful back to prevent potentially serious problems. Conservative therapeutic approaches include bed rest, medications, and mechanical support.

The back is a complex structure with multiple functions; it provides support for the basic bodily structure, protection for the spinal cord, and is integral in musculoskeletal motion. The biomechanics of the spine are extremely complex and require concise synchronization for proper function. Any alteration in the mechanical structure or surrounding tissues can lead to low back pain. There are numerous pain sensitive elements in the back including the vertebral body periosteum, the posterior longitudinal ligament, the synovium-lined facet joints, the nerve roots, and the paravertebral musculature. The paravertebral muscles respond to irritating stimuli by diffuse pain and reflex contractures. This muscle spasm frequently contributes to the painful back syndrome.

The complex nature of the back leads to numerous causes of back pain. These etiologies are diverse with different pathogenic mechanisms and therapeutic treatment options. Proper diagnosis is the most important factor so that a proper treatment plan can be developed. For example, a patient suffering from back pain secondary to compression by an abdominal aortic aneurysm will not respond to conservative management of bed rest, medications, and supporting braces. This extreme case exemplifies the importance of an accurate diagnosis. It is the physician's task to separate those individuals with potentially serious disease that require extensive diagnostic evaluation from the more common musculoskeletal pain often of unknown etiology.

If the initial diagnostic visit suggests no serious pathological or structural disease of the spine, nerves, cord or surrounding structures, then the patient should be treated with the diagnosis of lumbar strain. The pathophysiology of this condition is insufficiently understood and different treatment modalities are difficult to assess. Fortunately, most patients recover in a short period of time with reassurance and conservative management. Acute lumbar strain accompanied by severe pain is best managed by absolute bed rest, warm tub baths, heating pads, medications, firm mattress with a bed board, gentle physical massage, analgesics and rarely a corset or brace until the acute episode subsides. As the patient improves, gradual ambulation and physical therapy should be encouraged. An exercise program aimed at strengthening and stretching the paravertebral muscles should be initiated to decrease the chances of recurrent episodes.

Medications used in the treatment of low back pain have been controversial. Because most patients improve symptomatically over time, it is difficult to assess the efficacy of various therapeutic preparations. The drugs utilized in this condition include the skeletal muscle relaxants (e.g., carisoprodol (SOMA) and cyclobenzaprine (FLEXERIL)), nonsteroidal anti-inflammatory agents (e.g., aspirin, sulindac (CLINORIL) and indomethacin (INDOCIN)), and sedatives (e.g., phenobarbital and chloral hydrate (NOCTEC)). These medications should not be the sole form of therapy but rather as part of a therapeutic regimen. Sedatives are employed following the initial insult when the discomfort is severe, but should be quickly tapered after the initial episode. The skeletal muscle relaxants are useful when low back pain is accompanied by painful muscle spasm. Severe muscle spasm can act as a compressive force eliciting more pain and preventing rehabilitation. There are several spasmolytic compounds available in oral and parenteral forms. Nonsteroidal anti-inflammatory agents are effective when there is considerable tissue damage and edema, or to provide significant non-opioid analgesia. See Table N for proper dosages of skeletal muscle relaxants.

A small portion of patients will continue to have back pain following an extended period of conservative management. These patients may require further diagnostic evaluation to rule out serious disease. Consideration should be given to traumatic, metabolic, infectious, systemic, carcinomatous, and referred etiologies of low back pain. The majority of the evaluations will be negative and the patient's condition will be diagnosed as chronic lumbar strain. This is best managed with conservative treatment consisting of weight loss, postural correction, a firm mattress with bed board, and daily exercises to strengthen the lower back. Referral to a comprehensive pain management center may be appropriate for rehabilitation. However, like most disease states, the later the referral, the more difficult and less successful the treatment.

TRIGEMINAL NEURALGIA

Trigeminal neuralgia or tic douloureux is a common facial pain syndrome of unknown etiology. The disease is characterized by sudden, sharp high intensity facial pain in the distribution of one or more divisions of the trigeminal nerve. The distribution of pain most commonly involves the maxillary (V2) and/or mandibular branch (V3) of the trigeminal nerve, while sparing the ophthalmic branch (V1). Therefore, the pain usually affects the lower jaw or cheek region, and less often, the forehead. The pain occurs in brief bursts, usually lasting only a few seconds and is often followed by a refractory period, during which time pain is not experienced. However, during an attack of tic douloureux the pain frequently occurs in clusters of continuous pain for an extended duration.

Spontaneous remissions and exacerbations are common in the natural history of the disease and between attacks the patient is asymptomatic. Ninety percent of cases begin after the age of forty and women are affected more often than men. The brief, stabbing pain, is frequently precipitated by trigger zones located on the ipsilateral face or mouth and may be initiated by simple tasks such as eating, talking, or brushing teeth. The pain is so severe that some patients will go to extremes to avoid triggering attacks, including refusing to eat. Neurologic examination is normal in idiopathic trigeminal neuralgia and the diagnosis is based on a careful history. If the features typical of idiopathic tic douloureux are absent or altered, then the diagnosis should be questioned. In these cases, the physician must rule out causes of trigeminal irritation, such as tumor, multiple sclerosis, or brain stem infarct involving the trigeminal nerve tract.

The treatment of trigeminal neuralgia is difficult because the natural history dictates exacerbations and asymptomatic remissions. These remissions make therapeutic modalities difficult to compare in patients suffering from this condition. Also, patient compliance is difficult to maintain during the asymptomatic period for comparisons of different therapies. However, therapeutic options available to the physician and patient can be divided into medical and surgical approaches.

DRUG TREATMENT. Drug therapy for this disease consists of three primary agents: carbamazepine (TEGRETOL), phenytoin sodium (DILANTIN) and baclofen (LIORESAL). Tricyclic antidepressants may also be beneficial as an adjunctive treatment. Another compound reported to be effective is the skeletal muscle relaxant chlorphenesin carbamate (MAOLATE); however, further studies are required to establish its efficacy in this condition. True analgesic medications are not useful in the management of this condition because of the unpredictable onset and brief duration of the pain.

Carbamazepine (TEGRETOL) is the drug of choice and the most efficacious oral preparation. Therapy is initiated with 100 mg twice daily and the dose is gradually increased until relief is achieved or adverse effects are observed. The total daily dose generally should not exceed 1200 mg because of dose-related side effects including dizziness, sedation, and ataxia. However there are reports where as much as 3600 mg per day have been used. The patient may experience pain relief after the initial dose, but blood levels of 6 to 12 μg/mL are usually required to stop the lancinating pain. Serious idiosyncratic reactions such as aplastic anemia, platelet suppression, leukopenia, and abnormal liver function tests are rare, but require discontinuation of the drug if they occur. The patient must be monitored by complete biochemical and hematological profiles and must be followed at appropriate intervals to prevent the occurrence of potentially serious adverse effects.

Phenytoin sodium (DILANTIN) was the original anticonvulsant utilized for the treatment of trigeminal neuralgia. It is less effective than carbamazepine, but may be substituted in cases refractory to carbamazepine therapy. Phenytoin sodium may also be prescribed in patients unable to tolerate carbamazepine therapy. The dosage required for symptomatic control is 200 to 400 mg per day, orally, with dosages as high as 700 mg per day required on rare occasions, which will achieve therapeutic blood levels in the range of 10 to 20 μg/mL. Therapy with phenytoin sodium may also be discontinued secondary to dose-related adverse effects of sedation, nystagmus, and ataxia or idiosyncratic reactions of hepatitis, blood dyscrasias, gingival hypertrophy, and rashes. Patients treated with this drug should also be followed with blood chemistries at appropriate intervals.

Baclofen (LIORESAL) is the third agent utilized in the management of trigeminal neuralgia. This compound has shown efficacy in refractory cases of this condition and some physicians feel baclofen may be useful as an initial treatment modality, despite the fact that the Food and Drug Administration has not formally approved baclofen for this purpose. Therapy is initiated with 5 to 10 mg three times daily taken orally, and gradually increased to between 60 and 80 mg daily (or a mean dose of approximately 1 mg per kg). The most common side effects of baclofen are drowsiness, vomiting, and weakness. Chronic administration of this compound should not be followed by sudden withdrawal because of the potential for hallucinations, anxiety, and tachycardia.

SURGICAL TREATMENT. Much controversy surrounds the surgical treatment of trigeminal neuralgia. Surgery is utilized after a trial of medical therapy has failed or the patient has developed unacceptable side effects to the medications. Neurosurgeons differ in their surgical approaches to this condition and frequently patients are discouraged with the results. Many operative procedures are available and most consist of interruption of the trigeminal nerve pathway along its route. Glycerol rhizolysis is most commonly employed as the first line neurosurgical procedure of choice in the treatment of trigeminal neuralgia. When performed by experienced hands, it has a high success rate. The procedure involves placement of a needle under local anesthesia, sedation and monitored anesthetic care.

The most recent procedure advocated for treating trigeminal neuralgia is microsurgical decompression of the trigeminal root which extends between the ganglion and brain stem. The postulation supporting this procedure is that tic pain is due to pressure on the trigeminal root caused by tension of a nearby blood vessel. This intracranial operation is performed through a small posterior fossa craniotomy originating behind the ear. The trigeminal nerve root is exposed and microsurgical techniques separate the blood vessel and root. This technique requires expert skill and experience to decrease the potential complications of this major intracranial operation and offers the advantage of pain relief without producing significant changes in facial sensation.

PSYCHOLOGICAL CONSIDERATIONS IN THE MANAGEMENT OF CHRONIC PAIN SYNDROME

Pain is difficult to define. The specific description resides with medical findings and the subjective complaints and behaviors of the patient. Each incidence of pain must be analyzed in terms of the patient who is experiencing the pain. Individual tolerance and perceptions figure heavily in rating the degree of pain.

Pain varies with regard to duration, intensity, and impact upon the patient. The physician must combine medical findings with patient reports and observations of patient behaviors to fully assess the situation. As discussed previously, pain can be acute or chronic. Acute pain tends to be self-limiting and is generally thought to last no longer than 6 months. Chronic pain, however, is best defined as pain that exceeds the 6 month boundary and can last for months or years. Turk *et al.* (1983) cite three types of chronic pain:

Chronic Periodic Pain - this refers to acute episodes that occur intermittently over a period of time, e.g., vascular headache, trigeminal neuralgia.

Chronic Intractable Benign Pain - this pain is experienced consistently over time, but the intensity may vary.

Chronic Progressive Pain - this category is limited to pain associated with malignancies.

A number of patients who have chronic pain are able to adapt in a healthy manner, i.e., they encounter minimal disruption to their daily lives. However, a segment of chronic pain patients not only struggle with pain, but have the additional burden of experiencing a radical disruption in their daily lives. This dual impairment of pain and life disruption is referred to as *chronic pain syndrome*. This disorder has been further characterized with the following: (a) pain itself becomes the disease and serves no useful biological purpose; (b) depressed mood is observable; (c) opioids are iatrogenic due to the long standing nature of the pain; (d) drug dependence is likely due to over prescribing, multiple drug prescribing, or poor patient compliance with medications; and (e) cure or pain relief may not be feasible.

Due to its complexity and duration, the impact of chronic pain syndrome is far reaching, incorporating risks for the patient and the community. For example, the patient is at risk for limited life styles, including the potential for depression, overdose, drug dependence, and suicide. Health care systems are at risk when multiple interventions are to no avail. Societal risks are represented by the loss of contributing productive citizens who, instead, are disabled. Clearly it is advantageous for a variety of systems, including patient, family, health care, and society, to help the patient move from the confines of chronic pain syndrome to a less impaired position.

One method of understanding the psychological development, maintenance and therapeutic management of chronic pain syndrome is based upon a behavioral or operant conditioning model. Basically, this model, as proposed by Fordyce (1976), suggests that pain behavior is a learned response and therefore can be modified. The emphasis in this approach is to assess pain behavior, including motor, verbal and non-verbal behaviors (grimaces, listing, looking pained, etc.). A careful monitoring of antecedent (environmental triggers), behaviors (pain) and especially consequences (reinforcers for pain) are noted. The critical theme in the operant approach to understanding chronic pain is the interaction among environmental cues, pain behavior, and environmental reinforcers that follow pain behavior. In essence, the model attempts to define the circumstances wherein pain behavior occurs, and the resulting "pay-offs".

ASSESSMENT AND TYPES OF REINFORCEMENT

To understand the development and maintenance of chronic pain syndrome, the clinician needs to assess the response to pain:

Who is reinforcing pain behaviors?
When does this take place?
How is it done?
Where does this occur?
What behaviors in the patient signal pain?
How can the patterns be altered?

Reinforcement patterns are observable in patients and in their situations with family and others. These response patterns contribute to the development of chronic pain syndrome and must be addressed.

DIRECT AND POSITIVE REINFORCEMENT. According to Fordyce (1976), pain behavior may be maintained as a result of positive consequences following pain behavior. Often this will take the form of attention, concern and general nurturance, primarily from significant others, e.g., family, friends, and associates.

A clinical example is Ms. A., age 42, who was married to the same man for the past 23 years. This couple had four children and Ms. A remained home to care for their offspring. While she tended to the home, her husband worked diligently and at the age of 44 was promoted to Senior Vice-President of a major international corporation. Unfortunately, a price was paid for his diligence by his wife; she stated during the clinical interview that she felt neglected and abandoned by him for a number of years. At the age of 40, Ms. A developed a bulging disc at L5-S1. She was treated conservatively but with little subjective relief. Post therapy CT scans revealed a much improved picture, but her pain continued unabated. A series of visits to the home revealed the husband to be overly solicitous to his wife whenever she demonstrated pain. He would ask if he could do anything to make her more comfortable, frequently would bring her snacks or tea and, in general, would simply hold her hand and state, "I'm with you". Indeed, he even cancelled a number of business trips in order to insure her welfare. Two of the children who were away at college, eventually transferred to a local school so that they could be available to Ms. A on a day-to-day basis.

While Ms. A's pain initially may have been due to organic factors, the direct and positive reinforcement she received from her family likely maintained her painful status. Indeed when asked how her relationship with her husband changed as a result of her pain, she stated clearly, "He's like a new person, very attentive and caring". Further complicating the clinical picture was Ms. A's dependence on opioids, which either her husband or children provided to her on an "as needed" basis. Basically her complaints of pain resulted in the administration of nurturance and opioids. This reinforced her pain complaints and created and supported her drug dependence.

INDIRECT BUT POSITIVE REINFORCEMENT OF PAIN BEHAVIOR. This is referred to as behavior that has as its consequence, the avoidance of a painful situation. In order to be maintained, the behavior need not be successful all of the time, but only intermittently. Once established, an avoidance or protective behavior (e.g., limp, list, restriction in range of motion, dosage of analgesic medications, etc.) is difficult, though not impossible to modify. The avoidance behavior may have been appropriate and beneficial in the management of acute pain. However, unless modified, a chronic pain syndrome is likely to develop.

A clinical example is the case of Mr. B. He was employed as a laborer in a national chain of lumber supply stores for 15 years. One year prior to his injury he was promoted to a supervisory position. While his rate of pay increased considerably, he was now required to supervise, reprimand, and oversee his colleagues of many years. Mr. B stated in the clinical interview that he felt ambivalent about the position; he enjoyed the considerable increase in salary but despised the role of supervising his colleagues of many years. In addition, he felt they resented his ascent within the organization. As time passed he became more anxious, gained 25 pounds due to overeating, began to drink to excess, and experienced chronic sleep deficits. After 8 months on the job he slipped on the warehouse floor and the next morning could not get out of bed. A CT scan revealed a herniated disc at L4-L5 and L5-S1. Surgery was performed in addition to an active and progressive course of physical therapy. Despite the success of the therapeutic measures, Mr. B continued to complain of pain and an inability to return to his prior work. His employer was willing to structure a limited duty program, but Mr. B declined stating that the pain was too intense.

During one of the clinical interviews, Mr. B broke down and wept profusely, stating that he simply could not return to the supervisory position. He indicated that he did not have the skills to manage people, and as a result he felt abandoned by his colleagues and not accepted by the management. Mr. B's wife, in an independent interview, stated she felt he could have returned to work months ago, but that something was holding him back. She based her assessment on his ability to handle a series of ongoing household tasks requiring persistent physical activity.

After a period of time it became apparent that Mr. B's "pain" represented an effective avoidance of an even more painful situation, i.e., his work as a supervisor. Unfortunately, Mr. B's legal counsel, orthopedic expert witness, and substantial worker's compensation and eventual permanent disability payments precluded establishing a behavior intervention program. Mr. B was awarded total disability much to the astonishment of his orthopedic surgeons and the physical therapy team.

EXTINCTION OR PUNISHMENT OF WELL BEHAVIOR. In addition to the direct and indirect (avoidance) reinforcement of pain behaviors, the patient's environment can contribute to the chronic pain syndrome by discouraging or preventing well behavior. The usual players in this scenario are the patient and the family. For a myriad of reasons, the family may feel it is in the patient's, or their, best interest to maintain the patient in a dysfunctional state. This is done by admonishing the patient when they attempt an activity; a more skillful maneuver is to stay one step ahead and complete tasks prior to the patient having the opportunity to engage in them.

A clinical example involves Ms. C who was an active police officer employed by a major metropolitan city. She was 38 years old, married for 16 years with two children and had been an officer for 14 years. She had been cited for heroism twice by the police commissioner and clearly was rising within the organization. She described one evening after grocery shopping, leaning into the trunk of her automobile to pick up packages, and felt "something pull in my back". By the next afternoon she could not exit her squad car and had to be transported to the nearest hospital emergency room. A series of imaging techniques revealed herniated discs at L4-L5 and L5-S1. That night she had pain and lost bowel and bladder control. An operation was performed and deemed a success by both the surgeons and patient. She regained control of bodily functions and the pain had reduced considerably. Physical therapy assessed the patient as quite involved in her care; she was discharged with an 8 week leave from her job. Five weeks later, psychological consultation was requested by her surgeon since the patient seemed to be depressed and lacking in motivation. A review of her psychological profile revealed depression and helplessness. Numerous home visits portrayed the following behavioral dynamic: whenever the patient attempted any activity that required effort and mobility, her husband or another relative would engage the task and complete it. A meeting with the husband and relatives involved elicited that care and concern for the patient was one motivating force behind these maneuvers. When pressed, the husband also acknowledged his concern and worry regarding the inherent dangers of his wife's work. A series of family meetings were held, the dynamics of control and vulnerability were revealed, and within a short period of time the husband and patient began to work in a collaborative relationship to increase her independence, mobility, and strength. Behaviorally, the primary patient turned out to be the patient's family system, which inhibited her access to well behaviors. Within 4 weeks the patient returned to limited duty status and by 10 weeks had resumed full duty.

INTERVENTION TECHNIQUES AND STRATEGIES

In planning for an appropriate intervention, the practitioner will need to establish for the patient: (a) the pain related behaviors which occur frequently and need to be reduced; (b) the well behavior which occur infrequently or not at all and need to be increased; and (c) the behavioral skills level of the patient and the ability to attain reasonable goals.

A variety of simple techniques can be utilized to gather data, to assess the pain related patterns, to establish a measurement scale for pain for the individual, and to analyze the impact upon daily life. In the data collection processes, the behaviors, and the individual's supporting pain, become evident. With these facts in place, intervention plans can be formulated. The assessment tool can then be further utilized to track the success of the interventions.

CLINICAL INTERVIEWS

With regard to pain behaviors, the who, what, when, etc. are best addressed in clinical interviews with the patient and significant others. These interviews can involve the patient only, the significant others only, or a combination of both parties. Basically the task for the clinician is to determine the profile of pain behaviors (who, what, etc.), and assess what the significant others do to either reinforce pain behaviors or reduce the opportunities for well behavior. The task is to collect data, make observations, and identify recurring patterns.

DAILY ACTIVITY DIARY

The patient should be provided with a daily activity diary wherein activities are charted on an hourly basis. Basically the diary allows quick access to how much time was spent in "uptime" activities, i.e., non-reclining behaviors, versus "downtime" or reclining behavior. The diary can be designed to include notations for environmental cues, behavior and consequences. The diary also allows for investigation as to what circumstances provoke pain versus providing relief; also helpful is the rating of pain on a numerical scale.

The above activities are designed to alter the consequences of the patient's behavior. In essence, pain behaviors are now to be ignored by the significant others and uptime behaviors are to be reinforced. This is always done on a gradual basis with a rationale presented to both the patient and significant others. It is also helpful to have the patients and their families describe activities that were enjoyed prior to a painful lifestyle, and to assess the probability of designing a structure that would allow access to this pleasure and improve the quality of life.

MEDICATION REVIEW

The issue of medication needs to be addressed since many patients with chronic pain syndrome are dependent on their pain medication. As a result they may increase their tolerance and flirt with toxicity. Frequently, medication is taken or provided to the patient by significant others on an "as needed" (prn) basis, which is often defined by the patient as the first perception of pain.

The "pain cocktail" intervention helps to reduce the medication required for the management of pain. Initially, a baseline level of all pain medications is taken on a daily basis and recorded. This amount of drug(s) becomes the ingredients in a "cocktail" which uses a taste-masking vehicle such as cherry syrup. The cocktail is then taken on a fixed schedule, regardless of whether the patient feels he (or she) requires it. In this manner, medication becomes time-contingent rather than pain-contingent. The taste-masking vehicle allows for a gradual decrease in the active ingredient(s) over the course of treatment.

AVOIDANCE MANAGEMENT

As mentioned previously, if pain behaviors provide a means of escaping or avoiding other more painful situations, the issue will need to be addressed. If pain allows for the avoidance of family or social gatherings, brief psychotherapy or skill development may be needed. If pain awards intimacy and supports sexual dysfunction, brief treatment emphasizing communication skills or sex therapy may be in order.

COGNITIVE BEHAVIORAL INTERVENTIONS

The emphasis within this approach is that our thoughts can either enhance or diminish the experience of pain. Basically the emphasis is to be the support of the patient with a coping model of behavior which is problem-solving focused. Patient goals are determined by the patient, significant others and health professionals. These goals are further defined as short term, intermediate term, and long term. The initial goals often include reduction in medication, increase in "uptime" behaviors and decrease in "downtime" behaviors. Graded exercise and activities are structured with inputs from physicians and physical therapists. Frequently the psychologist will work with the patient's internal self-statements, e.g., "I'm in pain and need to rest". Alternatives are developed, e.g., "I'm in pain; I'll do a less strenuous activity". The goal is to change a life style that is controlled and driven by pain to one that is active, productive and self-enhancing.

Turk and Andy (1992) recently elaborated upon cognitive constructs as they apply to chronic pain. They included the following three components: (a) *cognitive schema* — general beliefs, appraisals, and expectations regarding pain; (b) *cognitive processes* — mental processes in attempts at pain control; and (c) *cognitive content* about specific patient circumstances and their attempts to cope with pain.

With regard to cognitive schema, the patient's processing of information related to his/her disease, management, prognosis, etc., may have aa direct effect upon the anxiety, depression, motivation, and life outlook. If every pain episode is viewed as potentially life-threatening, the general response is likely quite different from that of the person who views the pain as unfortunate, but manageable. Our cognitive assessments of pain events can either heighten the perception of pain and consequent behavioral dysfunction, or divert our attention from the perception of pain. Also, our anticipation of outcomes can influence behavior. If a patient cognitively anticipates exercise will lead to pain, he/she is less likely to engage in exercise. However, if exercise is anticipated to decrease future episodes associated with pain, the patient is more likely to exercise.

With respect to cognitive process, we know a significant number of chronic pain patients carry the additional burden of depression. Depressed affect is likely due to reduced activity as well as cognitive distortions. Cognitive distortions may include negative self statements, negative thoughts regarding social interaction and expectation, and self blame.

Cognitive content can be conceptualized as how the patient actively manages the impact of pain in their lives, i.e., how they cope. Coping strategies influence the self regulation of pain, and, in turn, the ability to measure and tolerate pain.

PROBLEM SOLVING STRATEGIES. These are taught as a means of enhancing productivity and independence. The emphasis is upon stating the problem clearly and the development of alternative responses. Each alternative is assessed with regard to its potential positive and negative aspects. Further elaboration as to the probability of those aspects is also made. Based upon these assessments, effective problem solving can be implemented.

RELAXATION RESPONSE. The patient who experiences pain frequently is tense, which further increases pain. Many patients have found the relaxation response to be an effective pain reducer. There are a number of methods for inducing the relaxation response, including deep breathing and imagery. With deep breathing, the goal is to consciously reduce the number of breaths taken. Each inhalation is thought of as an occasion to cleanse the body, while exhalation is viewed as an opportunity to reduce pain to manageable levels. With imagery, the patient is instructed to develop three images, based upon real experiences that provoke a sense of peacefulness. The temporal aspects of each scene can be related to any time period, from the present to childhood. The patient is asked to write two paragraphs describing each scene. Included in a scene are variables such as color, touch, smell, sound, etc. The patient is to actively project himself, or herself, into the image and to vicariously experience it. Essentially the patient is being provided with a cognitive strategy that will counteract pain. Not only is the patient not concentrating on the pain but he, or she, is cognitively removed from it.

METHODS OF MEASURING PAIN

Pain, is a very subjective phenomenon, and does not lend itself to be quantitated accurately. Physicians are taught to interview patients with pain by asking the standard historical questions of pain onset, location, duration, frequency, and radiation. Some idea of the quality and intensity of the pain is obtained by asking the patient whether the pain is sharp, dull, crampy, etc., and whether it is mild, moderate or severe. Attempts to ask the patient to describe the pain himself or herself by asking such open-ended questions as "Tell me what you are feeling now." are, at times, much more useful, but unfortunately, are often hampered by the patient's inability to express his/her pain experience to the physician in a meaningful way. Nonetheless, this traditional pain interview approach is usually sufficient in an acute situation to provide the physician with adequate information to formulate a reasonable differential diagnosis. However, this traditional approach is of little help when the physician is required to evaluate analgesic responsiveness in chronic pain syndromes, or to assess analgesic efficacy of new agents in clinical trials. In these two special situations, the physician must have a more quantitative means of evaluating pain intensity so that temporal comparisons could be made. Three techniques commonly employed in such situations are described below.

NUMERICAL SCALE. The simplest method for quantifying pain is asking the patient to rate his/her pain on a four point scale of 0, 1, 2, or 3. Often words such as *none*, *slight*, *moderate* and *severe* are associated with these numbers so the patient can better relate the numbers to a subjective experience. While this technique is quick, simple, and proven reliable in the single dose evaluation of analgesic efficacy in clinical trials, it may not be sensitive enough to evaluate the daily status of pain in chronic pain patients nor the overall response to treatment. Two other approaches may allow the patient the ability to better express his/her current status or, more helpful, allow assessment of the patient's overall response to treatment. A scale of 0 to 5 may be used as follows: 0 = no pain, 1 = mild pain , 2 = discomforting pain, 3 = distressing pain, 4 = horrible pain, and 5 = excruciating pain, limiting to constant bed rest. This system while very simple and easily understood by all patients, provides more than enough information to guide treatment and therapeutic plans. However, if more information is required (e.g., research purposes), a modification of the McGill Pain Questionnaire may be utilized. The patient is asked to rate his/her pain numerically on a scale of 1 to 10, with 1 being equivalent to pain that is just barely perceptible, and 10 being pain so excruciating that one would rather die than continue in such pain. As a means of assessing the patient's tolerance for pain, he/she is asked to rate in a similar way the pains from his/her worst toothache, headache, stomach ache, kidney stone, or if female, labor pain.

VISUAL ANALOG SCALE. The visual analog scale of pain quantitation is similar to a numerical scale in that the patient quantitates subjectively one aspect of his/her pain experience, usually intensity. However, instead of choosing a number, the subject is asked to mark a point on a line usually labeled as "no pain" on one end and "worse possible pain" at the other end. The line is then divided into ten equal spaces and the interval that contains the subject's mark is then given a value of 1 to 10. Although slightly more difficult to administer then the verbal numerical method, some investigators feel that the visual analog scale is a more accurate technique for pain measurement.

McGILL PAIN QUESTIONNAIRE. The use of either the numerical method or the visual analog scale for the evaluation of pain states assumes that a person's perception of pain is only related to its intensity, which changes in a linear fashion. In order to overcome these obvious limitations, some investigators have formulated multidimensional pain scales. The most popular method in this category is the McGill Pain Questionnaire (Fig. 5).

Subjects are given 20 word sets that describe a different dimension of pain and they are asked to select words relevant to their pain from each set. The questionnaire measures three aspects of the pain experience: sensory, affective and evaluative. Although difficult to administer and grade, the questionnaire has demonstrated characteristic response patterns for different pain syndromes such as cancer pain, lower back pain, arthritis, etc. The exact role of the McGill Pain

What Does Your Pain Feel Like?

Some of the words below describe your **present** pain. Circle ONLY those words that best describe it. Leave out any category that is not suitable. Use only a single word in each appropriate category-the one that applies best.

1	2	3	4
Flickering	Jumping	Pricking	Sharp
Quivering	Flashing	Boring	Cutting
Pulsing	Shooting	Drilling	Lacerating
Throbbing		Stabbing	
Beating		Lancinating	
Pounding			
5	**6**	**7**	**8**
Pinching	Tugging	Hot	Tingling
Pressing	Pulling	Burning	Itching
Gnawing	Wrenching	Scalding	Smarting
Cramping		Searing	Stinging
Crushing			
9	**10**	**11**	**12**
Dull	Tender	Tiring	Sickening
Sore	Taut	Exhausting	Suffocating
Hurting	Rasping		
Aching	Splitting		
Heavy			
13	**14**	**15**	**16**
Fearful	Punishing	Wretched	Annoying
Frightful	Grueling	Blinding	Troublesome
Terrifying	Cruel		Miserable
Vicious			Intense
Killing			Unbearable
17	**18**	**19**	**20**
Spreading	Tight	Cool	Nagging
Radiating	Numb	Cold	Nauseating
Penetrating	Drawing	Freezing	Agonizing
Piercing	Squeezing		Dreadful
	Tearing		Torturing

FIGURE 5. *Modified McGill Pain Questionnaire. (from Melzack, R.: "The McGill Pain Questionnaire: Major Properties and Scoring Methods," Pain* ***1****: 277 (1975).*

Questionnaire in the evaluation of acute and chronic pain syndromes is still actively being investigated.

CHRONIC ILLNESS PROBLEM INVENTORY (CIPI). This instrument consists of a paper and pencil test designed to assess behavioral problems associated with a myriad of chronic illnesses. The CIPI contains 65 items and yields 19 subscales. Each statement describes a problem in functioning, and the patient rates its applicability to it via a 5 point scale. The CIPI scales include activities of daily living, inactivity, social activity, contact with family and friends, employment, sleep, eating, finances, medication, thought processes, physical appearance, body deterioration, sex, assertion, medical interaction, marital overprotection, marital difficulty, and non-married relationships.

WEST HAVEN-YALE MULTIDIMENSIONAL PAIN INVENTORY (MPI). The MPI contains 52 items and yields 13 scales sorted into three major divisions. The instrument is designed to assess chronic pain as it results to cognitive-behavioral interventions. The first division measures the patients perception of pain intensity, affective disturbance, control, interference, and social support. The second division assesses the perception of the patient with regard to how significant others behave in the face of pain behavior displayed. The final division assesses general level of activity.

Research with the MPI has yielded three distinct subgroups of patients. The *dysfunctional* group score high on pain severity, life influence due to pain and increased psychological distress due to decrease in daily activities and perceptions of dyscontrol. The second group, referred to as *interpersonally distressed*, conceived their family and significant others as non-supportive. The final group, i.e., the *minimizes/adaptive copies*, had lower rating of pain severity, disruption of their lives, and affective distress. Additionally they endorsed items reflecting higher activity and increased control.

REFERENCES

------- "Rheumatology," In: *MKSAP VII Syllabus*, American College of Physicians, 1985, pp. 111-139.

------- "Transdermal Fentanyl," *The Medical Letter* **34** (Issue 881): 97-98 (1992).

Arnoff, G.M. (Ed.): *Evaluation and Treatment of Chronic Pain*, Urban and Schwarzenberg, Baltimore, 1985.

Augustinsson, L.E., C.A. Carlsson, and M. Fall: "Autonomic Effects of Electrostimulation," *Appl. Neurophysiol.* **45**: 185-189 (1982).

Augustinsson, L.E., C.A. Carlsson, J. Holm, and L. Jivegard: "Epidural Electrical Stimulation in Severe Limb Ischemia," *Ann. Surgery* **202**: 104-110 (1985).

Barolat, G., R.L. Knobler, and F.D. Lublin: "Trigeminal Neuralgia in a Patient with Multiple Sclerosis Treated with High Cervical Spinal Cord Stimulation," *Appl. Neurophysiol.* **51**: 333-337 (1988).

Barolat, G., J.B. Myklebust, and W. Wenninger: "Effects of Spinal Cord Stimulation on Spasticity and Spasms Secondary to Myelopathy," *Appl. Neurophysiol.* **51**: 29-44 (1988).

Barolat, G., J.B. Myklebust, and W. Wenninger: "Enhancement of Voluntary Motor Function Following Spinal Cord Stimulation - Case Study," *Appl. Neurophysiol.* **49**: 307-314 (1986).

Bechtel, T., and P.T. Pan: "When is TENS Effective and Practical for Pain Relief?," *J. Musculoskel. Med.* **2**: 37-43 (1985).

Bond, M.R.: Pain: *Its Nature, Analysis and Treatment*, Churchill Livingstone, New York, 1984.

Brechner, V.L., T. Ferrer-Brechner, and G.D. Allen: "Anesthetic Measures in Management of Pain Associated with Malignancy," *Semin. Oncol.* **4**: 99-108 (1977).

Brena, S.F., and W.D. Hammonds: "Nerve Blocks: Chemical and Deep Stimulation Analgesia," In: *Management of Patients with Chronic Pain*, Brena, S.F., and S.L. Chapman (Eds.), Spectrum Publications, New York, 1983, pp. 195-203.

Broseta, J., P. Roldan, J. Gonzalez-Darder, V. Bordes, and J.L. Barcia-Salorio: "Chronic Epidural Dorsal Column Stimulation in the Treatment of Causalgia Pain," *Appl. Neurophysiol.* **45**: 190-194 (1982).

Caldwell, J.R.: "Contemporary Management of Common Arthritic Diseases," *Compr. Ther.* **7**: 13-17 (1981).

Cedarbaum, J.M., and L.S. Schleifer: "Drugs for Parkinson's Disease, Spasticity, and Acute Muscle Spasms," In: *The Pharmacological Basis of Therapeutics, Eighth Edition*, Gilman, A.G., T.W. Rall, A.S. Nies, and P. Taylor (Eds.), Macmillan, New York, 1990, pp. 463-484.

De La Porte, C., and J. Siegfried: "Lumbosacral Spinal Fibrosis (Spinal Arachnoiditis). Its Diagnosis and Treatment by Spinal Cord Stimulation," *Spine* **8**: 593-603 (1983).

Delfino, U.: "An Advance in Trigeminal Therapy," In: *Persistent Pain: Modern Methods of Treatment, Volume 4*, Sampson, L., and J. Miles (Eds.), Grune and Stratton, New York, pp. 145-157 (1983).

Dimitrijevic, M.R., A.M. and Sherwood: "A System for Epidural Spinal Cord Stimulation," *Appl. Neurophysiol.* **45**: 465-467 (1982).

Dimitrijevic, M.R., et al.: "Spinal Cord Stimulation for the Control of Spasticity in Patients with Chronic Spinal Cord Injuries," *CNS Trauma* **3**: 129-144 (1986).

Downing, J.E., E.H. Busch, and P.M. Stedman: "Epidural Morphine Delivered by a Percutaneous Epidural Catheter for Outpatient Treatment of Cancer Pain," *Anesth. Analg.* **67**: 1159-1161 (1988).

Drechsel, U.: "Treatment of Cancer Pain with Neurolytic Agents," *Recent Results Cancer Res.* **89**: 137-147 (1984).

Fiume, D.: "Spinal Cord Stimulation in Peripheral Vascular Pain," *Appl. Neurophysiol.* **46**: 290-294 (1983).

Foley, K.M.: "The Rational Use of Analgesics in the Management of Patients with Acute and Chronic Pain," *Clin. Neurosurg.* **35**: 360-384 (1989).

Foley, K.M.: "The Treatment of Cancer Pain," *New Engl. J. Med.* **313**: 84-95 (1985).

Fordyce, W.E.: "Behavioral Methods for Chronic Pain and Illness," In: *The Psychology of Pain*, Sternbach, R.A. (Ed.), Raven Press, New York, 1986.

Hansten, P.D.: "Nonsteroidal Anti-inflammatory Drugs and Oral Anticoagulants," *Drug Interactions Newsletter* **3**: 49 (1983).

Hecker, B.R., L. and Albert: "Patient-controlled Analgesia: A Randomized Prospective Comparison Between Two Commercially Available PCA Pumps and Conventional Analgesic Therapy for Postoperative Pain," *Pain* **35**: 115-120 (1988).

Houde, R.W.: "Methods for Measuring Clinical Pain in Humans," *Acta Anaesth. Scand. (Suppl.)* **74**: 25-29 (1982).

Judkins, K.C., and M. Harmer: "Haloperidol as an Adjunct Analgesic in the Management of Post Operative Pain," *Anaesthesia* **37**: 1118-1120 (1982).

Kames, L.D., B.D. Naliboff, R.L. Heinrich, and C. Coscarelli-Schag: "The Chronic Illness Problems Inventory: Problem-oriented Psychological Assessment of Patients with Chronic Illness," *Int. J. Psych. Med.* **14**: 65-75 (1984).

Keats, A.S.: "The Effect of Drugs on Respiration in Man," *Annu. Rev. Pharmacol. Toxicol.* **25**: 41-65 (1985).

Keefe, F.V., J. Dunsmore, and R. Burnett: "Behavioral and Cognitive-Behavioral Approaches to Chronic Pain: Recent Advances and Future Directions," *J. Consult. Clin. Psychol.* **60**: 528-536 (1992).

Kerns, R.D., D.C. Turk, and T.E. Rudy: "TheWest Haven-Yale Multidimensional Pain Inventory (WHYMPI)," *Pain* **23**: 345-356 (1985).

Laska, E.M., A. Sunshine, F. Mueller, et al.: "Caffeine as an Analgesic Adjuvant," *J. Am. Med. Assoc.* **251**: 1711-1718 (1984).

Law, J.D.: "Failed Back Syndrome," *Joint Section on Spinal Disorders, 2nd Annual Meeting*, February 19-22, 1986, San Diego, CA.

Loeser, J.D., and K.J. Egan (Eds.): *Managing the Chronic Pain Patient. Theory and Practice at the University of Washington Multidisciplinary Pain Center*, Raven Press, New York, 1989.

Martin, R., Y. Lamarche and J.P. Tetrault: "Epidural and Intrathecal Narcotics," *Can. Anaesth. Soc. J.* **30**: 662-673 (1983).

Meglio, M., and B. Cioni: "Personal Experience with Spinal Cord Stimulation in Chronic Pain Management," *Appl. Neurophysiol.* **45**: 195-200 (1982).

Melzack, R.: "The McGill Pain Questionaire: Major Properties and Scoring Methods," *Pain* **1**: 277, 1975.

Meyerson, B.A.: "The Role of Neurosurgery in the Treatment of Cancer Pain," *Acta Anaesth. Scand.* **74**: 109-113 (1982).

Miles, J.: "Trigeminal Neuralgia," In: *Persistent Pain: Modern Methods of Treatment, Volume 4*, Sampson, L., J. and Miles (Eds.), Grune and Stratton, New York, pp. 223-247, 1983.

Nepomuceno, C., E. Faught, and K. Langford: "Diagnosis and Management of Low Back Pain," *Ala. J. Med. Sci.* **25**: 430-435 (1988).

Osterweis, M., A.K. Kleinman, and D. Mechanic (Eds.): *Pain and Disability: Clinical Behavioral and Public Policy Perspectives*, National Academy Press, Washington, D.C., 1987.

Porges, P.: "Local Anesthetics in the Treatment of Cancer Pain," *Recent Results Cancer Res.* **89**: 127-136 (1984).

Portenoy, R.K. K.M. and Foley: "Clinical and Pharmacological Considerations in the Use of Narcotic Analgesics in the Elderly," *Geriat. Med. Today* **4**: 32 (1985).

Posner, J.B.: "Disorders of Sensation," In: *Cecil's Textbook of Medicine, Volume 2*, Wyngaarden, J.B., and L.H. Smith (Eds.), W.B. Saunders, Philadelphia, 1985, pp. 2047-2064.

Reuler, J.B., D.E. Girard, and D.A. Nardone: "The Chronic Pain Syndrome: Misconceptions and Management," *Ann. Intern. Med.* **93**: 588-596 (1980).

Siegfried, J., A. Kuhner, and V. Sturm: "Neurosurgical Treatment of Cancer Pain," In: *Pain in the Cancer Patient*, Zimmermann, M., P. Drings, and G. Wagner (Eds.), Springer-Verlag, New York, 1984, pp. 148-156.

Simon, J.M.: "A Multidisciplinary Aproach to Chronic Pain," *Rehabil. Nurs.* **14**: 23-28 (1989).

Sriwatanakul, K., W. Kelvie, L. Lasagna, J.F. Calimlim, O.F. Weis, and G. Mehta: "Studies with Different Types of Visual Analog Scales for Measurement of Pain," *Clin. Pharmacol. Ther.* **34**: 234-239 (1983).

Stambaugh, J.E., and C. Lane: "Analgesic Efficacy and Pharmacokinetic Evaluation of Meperidine and Hydroxyzine, Alone and in Combination," *Cancer Invest.* **1**: 111-117 (1983).

Steardo, L., A. Leo, and E. Marano: "Efficacy of Baclofen in Trigeminal Neuralgia and Some Other Painful Conditions," *Eur. Neurol.* **23**: 51-55 (1984).

Swerdlow, M.: "Anticonvulsant Drugs and Chronic Pain," *Clin. Neuropharmacol.* **7**: 51-82 (1984).

Tonelli, L., T. Setti, A. Falasea, E. Martignon, E. Torcia, F.M. Calcaterra, G.A. Merli, and f. Facchinetti: "Investigation on Cerebrospinal Fluid Opioids and Neurotransmitters Related to Spinal Cord Stimulation," *Appl. Neurophysiol.* **51**: 324-332, 1988.

Turk, D.C., and T.E. Rudy: "Cognitive Factors and Persistent Pain: A Glimpse into Pandora's Box. *Cognit. Therap. Res.* **16**: 99-122 (1992).

Turk, D.C., D. Meichenbaum, and M. Genest: "Pain and Behavioral Medicine: A Cognitive Behavioral Perspective," In: *Chronic Pain*, France, R.D., and K.R.R. Krishnan (Eds.), American Psychiatric Press, Washington, D.C., 1988.

Wall, P.D., and R. Melzack (Eds.): *Textbook of Pain, Second Edition*, Churchill Livingstone, New York, 1989.

Walsh, T.D.: "Antidepressants in Chronic Pain," *Clin. Neuropharmacol.* **6**: 271-295 (1983).

Waltz, J.M., et al.: "Spinal Cord Stimulation and Motor Disorders Presentation," *5th International Congress on Biostimulation*, June 19-21, 1986, Monaco.

Wyant, G.M.: "Chronic Pain: Principles and Treatment," *Drugs* **26**: 262-267 (1983).

SELECTED DRUG INTERACTIONS

Several of the analgesics and adjuvants interact with other drugs, altering their pharmacokinetic properties and plasma levels. Thus, the therapeutic effectiveness and degree of toxicity of these drugs may be increased or reduced. The physician must be aware of any potential drug interactions when prescribing more than one agent, and should adjust the dose and dosage interval of each drug accordingly. A list of selected drug interactions is presented in this section.

DRUG COMBINATIONS	POTENTIAL EFFECT
Acetaminophen	
plus anticholinergics	Decreased acetaminophen absorption
plus barbiturates	Reduced acetaminophen effect; increased toxicity of acetaminophen overdose
plus cholestyramine	Decreased acetaminophen absorption
plus diazepam	Decreased diazepam bioavailability
plus ethanol	Chronic ethanol causes increased toxicity of acetaminophen overdose
plus food	Delayed acetaminophen absorption
plus metoclopramide	Increased acetaminophen absorption
plus oral contraceptives	Increased acetaminophen glucuronidation and increased plasma levels of ethinyl estradiol
plus phenytoin	Increased hepatic metabolism of acetaminophen
Amphetamines	
plus acetazolamide	Enhanced amphetamine effect
plus guanethidine	Decreased guanethidine effect
plus monoamine oxidase inhibitors	Severe sympathetic crisis
plus tricyclic antidepressants	Enhanced amphetamine effect

DRUG COMBINATIONS	POTENTIAL EFFECT
Antidepressants, tricyclic	
plus amphetamines	Enhanced amphetamine effect
plus barbiturates	Decreased antidepressant serum levels
plus cimetidine	Increased antidepressant toxicity
plus clonidine	Increased blood pressure
plus guanethidine	Increased blood pressure
plus propoxyphene	Increased antidepressant serum levels
Benzodiazepines	
plus cimetidine	Increased benzodiazepine serum levels
plus ethanol	Additive sedative effect
plus oral contraceptives	Increased and/or decreased benzodiazepine effect
Carbamazepine	
plus isoniazid	Increased carbamazepine toxicity
plus propoxyphene	Increased carbamazepine toxicity
plus theophylline	Decreased theophylline serum levels
plus warfarin	Decreased anticoagulant effect
Diflunisal	
plus aluminum containing antacids	Reduced diflunisal bioavailability
plus warfarin	Enhanced anticoagulant effect
Fenoprofen	
plus oral anticoagulants	Enhanced anticoagulant effect
Ibuprofen	
plus oral anticoagulants	Increased risk of bleeding

DRUG COMBINATIONS	POTENTIAL EFFECT
Indomethacin	
plus antacids	Decreased indomethacin absorption
plus β-adrenergic receptor blockers	Decreased antihypertensive effect
plus bumetanide	Decreased diuretic and antihypertensive effect
plus captopril	Decreased antihypertensive effect
plus corticosteroids	Increased incidence of gastrointestinal ulceration
plus furosemide	Decreased diuretic and antihypertensive effect
plus lithium carbonate	Increased lithium plasma levels
plus oral anticoagulants	Increased risk of bleeding
plus prazosin	Decreased antihypertensive effect
plus probenecid	Increased indomethacin plasma levels
plus thiazide diuretics	Mildly reduced antihypertensive effect
plus triamterene	Increased triamterene-induced nephrotoxicity
Ketoprofen	
plus methotrexate	Increased methotrexate toxicity
plus probenecid	Increased ketoprofen plasma levels
Meclofenamate	
plus warfarin	Increased anticoagulant effect
Mefanamic acid	
plus warfarin	Increased anticoagulant effect
Meperidine	
plus monoamine oxidase inhibitors	Increased adverse reactions (excitation, sweating, rigidity, and hypertension)
plus phenytoin	Reduced meperidine plasma levels
Methadone	
plus phenytoin	Reduced methadone plasma levels

DRUG COMBINATIONS	POTENTIAL EFFECT
Methotrimeprazine	
plus anticholinergics	Increased chance of anticholinergic symptoms
plus central nervous system depressants	Enhanced sedative effect
Naproxen	
plus oral anticoagulants	Increased risk of bleeding
plus probenecid	Increased naproxen plasma levels
Nonsteroidal anti-inflammatory drugs (NSAIDs)	
plus ACE-inhibitors	Reduced antihypertensive effects
plus β-adrenergic receptor blockers	Reduced antihypertensive effects
plus corticosteroids	Increased incidence of gastrointestinal ulceration
plus hydralazine	Reduced antihypertensive effects
plus prazosin	Reduced antihypertensive effects
Opioid analgesics	
plus barbiturates	Enhanced CNS depressant effects
plus cimetidine	Enhanced opioid effects
plus chlorpromazine	Enhanced CNS depression and hypotension
plus ethanol	Additive CNS depressant effects
plus neuromuscular blockers	Additive respiratory depression
plus rifampin	Decreased opioid plasma levels
Pentazocine	
plus smoking	Increased dosage requirement for pentazocine

DRUG COMBINATIONS	POTENTIAL EFFECT
Phenylbutazone	
plus methotrexate	Increased methotrexate toxicity
plus oral hypoglycemics	Enhanced hypoglycemic effect
plus warfarin	Enhanced anticoagulant effect
Phenytoin	
plus cimetidine	Enhanced phenytoin toxicity
plus disulfiram	Enhanced phenytoin toxicity
plus isoniazid	Enhanced phenytoin toxicity
plus phenylbutazone	Enhanced phenytoin toxicity
plus theophylline	Decreased theophylline serum levels
Piroxicam	
plus oral anticoagulants	Enhanced anticoagulant effect
Propoxyphene	
plus β-adrenergic receptor blockers	Increased propranolol and metoprolol plasma levels
plus carbamazepine	Increased carbamazepine toxicity
plus doxepin	Increased doxepin plasma levels
plus spironolactone	Increased incidence of spironolactone-induced gynecomastia
plus smoking	Increased dosage requirement for propoxyphene
Salicylates	
plus acetazolamide	Increased CNS toxicity of acetazolamide
plus ACE inhibitors	Decreased antihypertensive effect
plus antacids	Decreased salicylate plasma levels
plus cimetidine	Slightly increased salicylate plasma levels
plus corticosteroids	Increased salicylate elimination
plus ethanol	Enhanced aspirin-induced gastric mucosal damage and aspirin induced prolongation of bleeding time
plus heparin	Increased risk of bleeding
plus ketorolac	Increased ketorolac plasma levels
plus indomethacin	Increased indomethacin plasma levels

DRUG COMBINATIONS	POTENTIAL EFFECT
Salicylates (continued)	
plus methotrexate	Increased methotrexate toxicity
plus para-aminobenzoic acid (PABA)	Increased salicylate plasma levels
plus phenylbutazone	Increased uric acid plasma levels
plus probenecid	Reduced uricosuric effect of probenecid (analgesic doses of salicylates)
plus sulfinpyrazone	Reduced uricosuric effect of sulfinpyrazone (analgesic doses of salicylates)
plus sulfonylureas	Increased hypoglycemic effect
plus valproic acid	Increased free valproic acid plasma levels
Sulindac	
plus warfarin	Enhanced anticoagulant effect
Tolmetin	
plus oral anticoagulants	Increased risk of bleeding in anticoagulated patients

REFERENCES

Goldberg, K.E.: *Drug Interactions, Clinical Pocket Manual*, Nursing 88 Books, Springhouse Corp., Springhouse, 1988.

Hansten, P.D., and J.R. Horn: *Drug Interactions, 6th Edition*, Lea and Febiger, Philadelphia, 1989.

CONTROLLED SUBSTANCES ACT

The legal aspects of prescription writing and dispensing are incorporated in various federal, state and local laws, which the medical practitioner must understand and observe; the strictest law regardless of governmental level, always takes precedence unless Federal Law is preemptive. In 1970, the Comprehensive Drug Abuse Prevention and Control Act, commonly called the Controlled Substances Act, was signed into law. This act imposes even more stringent controls on the distribution and use of all stimulant and depressant drugs and substances with the potential for abuse as designated by the Drug Enforcement Administration (DEA), Department of Justice. This act divides drugs with abuse potential into five categories or schedules as follows:

Schedule I - Drugs in this schedule have a high potential for abuse and no currently accepted medical use in the United States. Examples of such drugs include heroin, marihuana, peyote, mescaline, some tetrahydrocannabinols, LSD, and a variety of opioid derivatives. Substances listed in this schedule are not for prescription use; they may be obtained for chemical analysis, research or instruction purposes by submitting an application and a protocol of the proposed use to the DEA.

Schedule II - The drugs in this schedule have a high abuse potential with severe psychological or physical dependence liability. Schedule II controlled substances consist of certain opioid drugs, preparations containing amphetamines or methamphetamines as the single active ingredient or in combination with each other, and certain sedatives. Examples of opioids included in this schedule are opium, morphine, codeine, alfentanil (ALFENTA), fentanyl (SUBLIMAZE), hydromorphone (DILAUDID), levorphanol (LEVO-DROMORAN), meperidine (DEMEROL), methadone (DOLOPHINE), cocaine, oxycodone (PERCODAN and TYLOX), oxymorphone (NUMORPHAN) and sufentanil (SUFENTA). Also included are stimulants, e.g., dextroamphetamine, methamphetamine, methylphenidate, and depressants, e.g., amobarbital, pentobarbital and secobarbital.

Schedule III - The drugs in this schedule have a potential for abuse that is less than for those drugs in Schedules I and II. The use or abuse of these drugs may lead to low or moderate physical dependence or high psychological dependence. Included in this schedule, for example, are glutethimide, methyprylon, phendimetrazine, and paregoric. Also some combination products containing codeine, e.g., EMPIRIN W/CODEINE, FIORINAL W/CODEINE, TYLENOL W/CODEINE.

Schedule IV - The drugs in this category have the potential for limited physical or psychological dependence and include barbital, phenobarbital, paraldehyde, ethchlorvynol, chloral hydrate, meprobamate, chlordiazepoxide, diazepam, clorazepate, flurazepam, oxazepam, clonazepam, prazepam, lorazepam, and propoxyphene (DARVON, DARVON-N, etc.).

Schedule V - Schedule V drugs have a potential for abuse that is less than those listed in Schedule IV. These consist of preparations containing moderate quantities of certain opioids for use in pain (i.e., buprenorphine (BUPRENEX)) or as antidiarrheals (e.g., diphenoxylate (LOMOTIL), difenoxin (MOTOFEN) or PAREPECTOLIN, which contains paregoric), or as antitussives (such as codeine-containing cough mixtures, e.g., ROBITUSSIN A-C). These may be dispensed without a prescription order in some States, provided that specified dispensing criteria are met by the pharmacist. For one of these to be considered a Schedule V preparation the preparation must contain:

1. not more than 200 mg of codeine per 100 mL or per gram.
2. not more than 100 mg of dihydrocodeine per 100 mL or per gram.
3. not more than 2.5 mg of diphenoxylate and not less than 25 ug of atropine sulfate per dosage unit.
4. not more than 0.5 mg of difenoxin and not less than 25 ug of atropine sulfate per dosage unit.
5. not more than 100 mg of opium per 100 ml or per gram.

Every person involved in the manufacture, importing, exporting, distribution or dispensing of any Controlled Drug must obtain an annual registration from the DEA; therefore, a physician must be registered before he/she can administer or dispense any of the drugs listed in the abuse schedules. Furthermore, the physician's DEA registration number must be indicated on every prescription order for Controlled Substances.

Renewal Information - The wishes of the prescriber with regard to refilling medication should be indicated on every prescription, and if renewals are authorized, the number of times. Prescription orders for drugs that bear the legend: "Caution: Federal laws prohibits dispensing without prescription" may not be refilled without the expressed consent of the prescriber. Prescriptions for drugs covered under Schedule III or IV of the Controlled Substances Act may be renewed, if so authorized, not more than five times within six months of date of issue; drugs within Schedule II may not be refilled.

MISCELLANEOUS DRUG TABLES

TABLE A. A STEPWISE APPROACH TO PAIN MANAGEMENT FOR SPECIFIC SYNDROMES

TYPE OF PAIN	INITIAL REGIMEN	IF RESPONSE IS INADEQUATE	IF RESPONSE IS STILL INADEQUATE
ACUTE PAIN			
Mild to moderate	Acetaminophen, aspirin or another NSAID	Add codeine, oxycodone, propoxyphene or pentazocine orally	Reevaluate the cause(s) of the pain
Severe	Parenteral opioids	Add parenteral hydroxyzine; increase the opioid dose, or add an NSAID if the patient can take oral medications; consider using a tricyclic antidepressant	Reevaluate the cause(s) of the pain
CHRONIC PAIN			
Benign	Acetaminophen, aspirin or another NSAID	Add analgesic adjuvants, or use an oral mixed agonist-antagonist opioid agent as infrequently as possible	Consider a neurosurgical or anesthetic procedure
Terminal, cancer related	Acetaminophen, aspirin or another NSAID with or without oxycodone, codeine, propoxyphene or pentazocine	Substitute oral morphine, hydromorphone, methadone or meperidine for the other oral opioid, or may consider use of fentanyl transdermal	Add parenteral opioids, epidural or intrathecal opioid infusion, or analgesic adjuvants

NSAID = nonsteroidal anti-inflammatory drug

TABLE B. POTENCY COMPARISONS OF SELECTED OPIOID ANALGESICS[a]

DRUG	EQUIANALGESIC DOSES (mg)		ORAL : PARENTERAL DOSE RATIO
	PO	IM	
AGONISTS			
Morphine	60	10	6.0
Codeine	200	120	1.7
Fentanyl	------[c]	0.1	------
Hydromorphone	7.5	1.5	5.0
Levorphanol	4	2	2.0
Meperidine	300	75	4.0
Methadone	20	10	2.0
Oxycodone	30	------[c]	------
Oxymorphone	10[d]	1	10.0
Propoxyphene	130	------[c]	------
Sufentanil	------[c]	0.02	------
MIXED AGONIST-ANTAGONISTS			
Buprenorphine	------[c]	0.3	------
Butorphanol	------[c]	2	------
Dezocine	------[c]	10	------
Nalbuphine	------[c]	10	------
Pentazocine	150	30	5.0

[a] The data in this Table are based upon morphine, 10 mg, administered intramuscularly and represent the general consensus of medical opinion. Variability will occur among patients; therefore, these values should be used only as a guide for comparison.

[b] These data were calculated as the ratio of the PO : IM equianalgesic doses of the compounds. The equianalgesic doses were estimated from dose-response curves and are based on the analgesic efficacy of the drugs. These data are not reflective of bioavailability which is based upon plasma concentrations of the drugs.

[c] Not used by this route.

[d] Rectal administration.

TABLE C. SOME PHARMACOKINETIC DATA OF OPIOID ANALGESICS

DRUG	ONSET OF EFFECT[a] (MINUTES)	PEAK EFFECT[a] (MINUTES)	DURATION OF EFFECT (HOURS)	PLASMA HALF-LIFE (HOURS)
AGONISTS				
Morphine	30	30 to 90	3 to 7	2 to 3
Alfentanil	------[b]	------------[b]	0.5 to 1	1 to 2
Codeine	30	45 to 90	4 to 6	3 to 4
Fentanyl	10	20 to 30	1 to 2	3 to 4
Hydromorphone	30	30 to 90	4 to 5	2 to 4
Levorphanol	30	60 to 90	4 to 8	10 to 12
Meperidine	15	30 to 60	2 to 4	3 to 4
Methadone	15	60 to 120	4 to 6	21 to 25
Oxycodone[c]	15	45 to 60	4 to 6	------------[b]
Oxymorphone	10	30 to 90	3 to 6	------------[b]
Propoxyphene[c]	60	60 to 90	4 to 6	6 to 12
Sufentanil	5	------------[b]	------------[b]	2 to 3
MIXED AGONIST-ANTAGONISTS				
Buprenorphine	15	45 to 60	4 to 6	2 to 3
Butorphanol	10	30 to 60	3 to 4	2 to 4
Dezocine	30	30 to 150	2 to 4	---------[b]
Nalbuphine	15	45 to 60	3 to 6	4 to 6
Pentazocine	15	30 to 60	2 to 3	2 to 3

[a] Based on intramuscular administration.

[b] No data available.

[c] Based on oral administration.

TABLE D. SELECTED INDIVIDUAL OPIOID ANALGESIC PREPARATIONS

GENERIC NAME	TRADE NAME	DOSAGE FORMS	COMMON ADULT DOSAGE	COMMON PEDIATRIC DOSAGE
Alfentanil Hydrochloride (C-II)	ALFENTA	**Inj:** 500 μg/mL	**Incremental Injection IV** **Procedures under 30 minutes duration:** For Induction, 8 - 20 μg/kg. For Maintenance, 3 - 5 μg/kg or 0.5 - 1 μg/kg/min. Total Dose, 8 - 40 μg/kg. **Procedures of 30 to 60 minutes duration:** For Induction, 20 - 50 μg/kg. For Maintenance, 5 - 15 μg/kg. Total Dose, up to 75 μg/kg. **Continuous Infusion IV** **Procedures of over 45 minutes duration:** For Induction, 50 - 75 μg/kg. For Maintenance, 0.5 - 3 μg/kg/min. Total Dose, dependent on the duration of the procedure. **Anesthetic Induction IV** **Procedures of over 45 minutes duration:** For Induction, 130 - 245 μg/kg. For Maintenance, 0.5 - 1.5 μg/kg/min. Total Dose, dependent on the duration of the procedure.	Not recommended for use in children under 12.
Buprenorphine Hydrochloride (C-V)	BUPRENEX	**Inj:** 0.324 mg/mL (equal to 0.3 mg/mL buprenorphine base)	**Pain:** 0.324 mg deep IM or slow IV (over 2 min) q 6 h prn. Repeat once, if needed, 30 - 60 min after initial dose.	Not recommended for use in children under 13.
Butorphanol Tartrate	STADOL	**Inj (per mL):** 1, 2 mg	**Pain:** 1 mg IV q 3 - 4 h prn or 2 mg IM q 3 - 4 h prn. **Anesthesia Premedication:** 2 mg IM 60 - 90 minutes before surgery. **Anesthesia Maintenance:** 0.5 - 1.0 mg IV (incremental dose).	Not recommended for use in patients under 18.

	STADOL NS	**Nasal Spray**: 10 mg/mL	**Pain**: 1 mg (1 spray in one nostril). May repeat in 30 - 60 min, if necessary.	Not recommended for use in patients under 18.
Codeine Sulfate (C-II)		**Tab**: 15, 30, 60 mg	**Pain**: 15 - 60 mg q 4 - 6 h po.	**Pain (over 1 year)**: 0.5 mg/kg q 4 - 6 h po.
Codeine Phosphate (C-II)		**Tab**: 30, 60 mg	**Pain**: 15 - 60 mg q 4 - 6 h po.	**Pain (over 1 year)**: 0.5 mg/kg q 4 - 6 h po.
		Inj (per mL): 30, 60 mg	**Pain**: 15 - 60 mg q 4 - 6 h IM, SC, or IV.	**Pain (over 1 year)**: 0.5 mg/kg q 4 - 6 h SC or IM.
Dezocine	DALGAN	**Inj (per mL)**: 5, 10, 15 mg	**Pain**: 5 - 20 mg q 3 - 6 h IM or 2.5 - 10 mg q 2 - 4 h IV.	Not recommended for use in patients under 18.
Fentanyl	DURAGESIC-25 DURAGESIC-50 DURAGESIC-75 DURAGESIC-100	**Transdermal**: rate = 25 μg/h **Transdermal**: rate = 50 μg/h **Transdermal**: rate = 75 μg/h **Transdermal**: rate = 100 μg/h	**Pain**: individualize based upon the status of the patient. Initially, use the 25 μg/h dose; may be worn on intact, clean, and dry skin for up to 72 h.	Not recommended for use in children.
Fentanyl Citrate (C-II)	SUBLIMAZE	**Inj**: 50 μg/mL (base equivalent)	**Anesthesia Premedication**: 50 - 100 μg/kg IM or slow IV 30 - 60 minutes prior to surgery. **Adjunct to General Anesthesia**: 2 - 20 μg/kg IV. Adjunct to Regional Anesthesia: 50 - 100 μg IM or slow IV. **Postoperatively**: 50 - 100 μg IM q 1 - 2 h prn.	**Anesthesia (Induction and Maintenance:** **Under 2 yrs**: Not recommended. **2-12 yrs**: 2 - 3 μg/kg IV.
Hydromorphone Hydrochloride (C-II)	DILAUDID	**Tab**: 2, 4, 8 mg **Oral Liquid**: 5 mg/5 mL **Rectal Suppos**: 3 mg **Inj (per mL)**: 1, 2, 4 mg	2 mg q 4 - 6 h po. 2.5 mg - 10 mg (2.5 - 10 mL) q 3 - 6 h po. 3 mg q 6 - 8 h rectally. 1 - 2 mg q 4 - 6 h SC or IM.	Safety and effectiveness in children have not been established.
	DILAUDID-HP	**Inj**: 10 mg/mL	1 - 2 mg q 4 - 6 h SC or IM.	Not recommended for use in children.
Levorphanol Tartrate (C-II)	LEVO-DROMORAN	**Tab**: 2 mg **Inj**: 2 mg/mL	2 mg q 6 - 8 h po. 2 mg q 6 - 8 h SC.	Not recommended for use in children.

GENERIC NAME	TRADE NAME	DOSAGE FORMS	COMMON ADULT DOSAGE	COMMON PEDIATRIC DOSAGE
Meperidine Hydrochloride (C-II)	DEMEROL	**Tab**: 50, 100 mg **Syrup**: 50 mg/5 mL	**Pain Relief**: 50 - 150 mg q 3 - 4 h po.	0.5 - 0.8 mg/lb q 3 - 4 h po.
		Inj (per mL): 25, 50, 75, 100 mg	**Pain Relief**: 50 - 150 mg q 3 - 4 h IM or SC. **Preoperative Medication**: 50 - 100 mg IM or SC 30 minutes before anesthesia. **Obstetrical Anesthesia**: 50 - 100 mg q 1 - 3 h IM or SC.	0.5 - 0.8 mg/lb q 3 - 4 h IM or SC 0.5 - 1.0 mg/lb IM or SC 30 to 90 minutes before anesthesia.
Methadone Hydrochloride (C-II)	DOLOPHINE	**Tab**: 5, 10 mg **Inj**: 10 mg/mL **Oral Solution (per 5 mL)**: 5, 10 mg	2.5 - 10 mg q 3 - 4 h po. 2.5 - 10 mg q 3 - 4 h IM or SC. 2.5 - 10 mg q 3 - 4 h po.	Not recommended for use in children.
	METHADONE HCL INTENSOL	**Oral Concentrate**: 10 mg/mL	2.5 - 10 mg q 3 - 4 h po.	
Morphine Sulfate (C-II)	------	**Tab**: 10, 15, 30 mg	5 - 30 mg q 4 h po.	Not recommended for use in children.
		Inj (per mL): 0.5, 1, 2, 3, 4, 5, 8, 10, 15 mg	**SC or IM**: 5 - 20 mg/70 kg q 4 h. **IV**: 2.5 - 15 mg/70 kg in 4 - 5 mL of Water for Injection, given over 4 - 5 min.	**SC or IM**: 0.1 - 0.2 mg/kg (up to 15 mg) q 4 h. **IV**: No information on use in pediatric patients under 18 years old is available.
		Drip: 30 mg in 150 mL D_5W	1 - 4 mg/h slow IV.	
	ASTRAMORPH PF, DURAMORPH	**Inj (per mL)**: 0.5, 1 mg	**IV Administration**: initial dose should be 2 - 10 mg/70 kg. **Epidural Administration**: a bolus dose of 5 mg in the lumbar region may provide satisfactory pain relief for up to 24 hours. If adequate pain relief is not achieved within 1 hour, careful administration of incremental doses of 1 to 2 mg at intervals sufficient to assess effectiveness may be given.	Not recommended for use in children. No information on use in pediatric patients under 18 years old is available.

			For continuous infusion, an initial dose of 2 - 4 mg per 24 hours is the recommendation. Further doses of 1 to 2 mg may be given if pain relief is not achieved initially. **Intrathecal Administration**: 0.2 - 1 mg may provide satisfactory pain relief for up to 24 hours.	No information on use in pediatric patients under 18 is available.
	MS CONTIN	**Controlled Release Tab**: 15, 30, 60, 100 mg	30 - 60 mg q 12 h po.	Not recommended for use in children.
		Inj (per mL): 0.5 to 15 mg	5 - 10 mg q 4 h SC or IM.	0.1 - 0.2 mg/kg q 4 h SC or IM.
	MSIR	**Oral Solution (per 5 mL)**: 10, 20 mg	5 - 30 mg q 4 h po.	Not recommended for use in children.
		Tab: 15, 30 mg	5 - 30 mg q 4 h po.	
	RMS	**Rectal Suppos**: 5, 10, 20, 30 mg	10 - 30 mg q 4 h rectally.	Not recommended for use in children.
	ROXANOL	**Rectal Suppos**: 5, 10, 20, 30 mg	10 - 30 mg q 4 h rectally.	Not recommended for use in children.
	ROXANOL ROXANOL 100	**Oral Solution**: 20 mg/5 mL **Oral Solution**: 100 mg/5 mL	10 - 30 mg q 4 h po. 10 - 30 mg q 4 h po.	Not recommended for use in children.
	ROXANOL RESCUDOSE	**Oral Solution**: 20 mg/5 mL	10 - 30 mg q 4 h po.	Not recommended for use in children.
	ROXANOL SR	**Sustained Release Tab**: 30 mg	30 mg q 8 h po.	Not recommended for use in children.
Nalbuphine Hydrochloride	NUBAIN	**Inj (per mL)**: 10, 20 mg	**Pain Relief**: 10 mg q 3 - 6 h SC, IM or IV. **Support to Balanced Anesthesia:** **Induction**: 0.3 - 3.0 mg/kg IV over 10 to 15 minutes. **Maintenance**: 0.25 - 0.50 mg/kg IV.	Not recommended for use in children.

GENERIC NAME	TRADE NAME	DOSAGE FORMS	COMMON ADULT DOSAGE	COMMON PEDIATRIC DOSAGE
Oxycodone Hydrochloride (C-II)	ROXICODONE	**Tab**: 5 mg	5 mg q 6 h po.	Not recommended for use in children.
	ROXICODONE INTENSOL	**Oral Solution**: 5 mg/5 mL	5 mg q 6 h po.	
Oxymorphone Hydrochloride (C-II)	NUMORPHAN	**Inj (per mL)**: 1, 1.5 mg	**Pain Relief**: 1 - 1.5 mg q 4 - 6 h SC or IM. **Preoperative Medication**: 1 - 1.5 mg SC or IM. **Obstetrical Anesthesia**: 0.5 - 1 mg IM.	Not recommended for use in children under 12.
		Rectal Suppos: 5 mg	**Pain Relief**: 5 mg q 4 - 6 h rectally.	Not recommended for use in children under 12.
Pentazocine Hydrochloride (C-IV)	TALWIN NX	**Tab**: 50 mg[1]	1 tab q 3 - 4 h po.	Not recommended for use in children under 12.
Pentazocine Lactate (C-IV)	TALWIN	**Inj**: 30 mg/mL (base equivalent)	30 mg q 3 - 4 h SC, IM or IV.	Not recommended for use in children under 12.
Propoxyphene Hydrochloride (C-IV)	DARVON	**Cpsl**: 32, 65 mg	65 mg q 4 h po.	Not recommended for use in children.
	DOLENE	**Cpsl**: 65 mg	65 mg q 4 h po.	Not recommended for use in children.
Propoxyphene Napsylate (C-IV)	DARVON-N	**Tab**: 100 mg	100 mg q 4 h po.	Not recommended for use in children.
		Oral Suspension: 50 mg/5 mL	100 mg q 4 h po.	Not recommended for use in children.

Sufentanil Citrate (C-II)	SUFENTA	**Inj**: 50 μg/mL (base equivalent)	**With Nitrous Oxide/Oxygen**: IV **Procedures of 1 - 2 hours duration**: For Induction, 1 - 2 μg/kg. For Maintenance, 10 - 25 μg/kg. **Procedures of 2 - 8 hours duration**: For Induction, 2 - 8 μg/kg. For Maintenance, 10 - 50 μg/kg. **With 100% Oxygen and a Muscle Relaxant**: IV use For Induction, 8 - 30 μg/kg. For Maintenance, 25 - 50 μg/kg.	Not recommended for use in children.

[1] Pentazocine tablets (TALWIN NX) also contain 0.5 mg naloxone to reduce the abuse potential.

(C-II): Schedule II, Controlled Substances Act.
(C-IV): Schedule IV, Controlled Substances Act.
(C-V): Schedule V, Controlled Substances Act.

TABLE E. APPROACH TO CLINICAL PROBLEMS ASSOCIATED WITH OPIOID USE

PROBLEM	RECOMMENDED THERAPY
Respiratory Depression	Use a mixed agonist-antagonist opioid; check arterial blood gases and monitor vital signs frequently.
Constipation	Administer stool softeners and/or irritant cathartics (see Table P).
Sedation	Use small doses of the opioid at more frequent intervals; consider the use of daytime central nervous system stimulants.
Drug Allergy	Use parenteral antihistamines (see Table P), treat anaphylaxis, or switch to an opioid of a different chemical structure.
Nausea and Vomiting	Switch to another opioid; coadminister an antiemetic drug, e.g., prochlorperazine.
Tolerance	Switch to another opioid.
Physical Dependence	Reduce the dose of the opioid gradually; switch to either a less potent compound or methadone and reduce the dose slowly.

TABLE F. SIGNS AND SYMPTOMS OF OPIOID WITHDRAWAL[a]

HOURS AFTER LAST DOSE	SIGNS AND SYMPTOMS[b,c]	
8 to 12	Lacrimation Rhinorrhea	Yawning Sweating
12 to 14	Restless ("Yen") Sleep	
18 to 20	Dilated Pupils Anorexia Gooseflesh Tremors	Restlessness Irritability Anxiety
48 to 72 (Peak)	Increased Irritability Insomnia Marked Anorexia Violent Yawning Severe Sneezing Lacrimation Coryza Muscle Spasms Generalized Body Aches	Nausea and Vomiting Diarrhea Abdominal Cramping Increased Heart Rate Increased Blood Pressure Chills and Hyperthermia Flushing Low Back Pain Hyperpnea

Duration of the withdrawal syndrome is approximately 7 to 10 days.

[a] For morphine and other mu receptor agonists with durations of action similar to morphine.

[b] The signs and symptoms of meperidine withdrawal usually begin to appear within 3 hours after the last dose, peak in 8 to 12 hours, and then decline; the duration is approximately 4 to 5 days. Lacrimation, rhinorrhea, sweating, pupillary dilation, nausea, vomiting and diarrhea are generally less severe than morphine; however, muscle spasms, restlessness, anxiety and irritability may be more intense.

[c] The methadone abstinence syndrome presents signs and symptoms similar to those listed above; however, the condition develops more slowly (24 to 48 hours after the last dose), is more prolonged (peak of 1 to 3 weeks; duration up to 6 to 7 weeks), and is usually less intense than the morphine withdrawal.

TABLE G. PHARMACOKINETIC DATA OF NON-OPIOID ANALGESICS

DRUG NAMES GENERIC AND (TRADE)	ORAL BIOAVAILABILITY (Percent)	TIME TO PEAK PLASMA CONC. (Hours)	ELIMINATION HALF-LIFE (Hours)	PLASMA PROTEIN BINDING (Percent)	VOLUME OF DISTRIBUTION (L/kg)	EFFECTIVE PLASMA CONCENTRATIONS (μg/mL)
Acetaminophen (TYLENOL, etc.)	90 to 100	0.5 to 1	2	20	0.80 to 1.00	10 to 20
Aspirin (ECOTRIN, EMPIRIN, etc.)	65 to 70	0.5 to 1	0.25 to 0.35[a]	80 to 90	0.15 to 0.20	20
Salicylic Acid	95 to 100	-------------[b]	2 to 3[a]	80 to 90	0.13 to 0.17	50 to 100
Diclofenac Sodium (VOLTAREN)	45 to 55	2 to 3	2	99	0.50 to 0.60	1 to 2
Diflunisal (DOLOBID)	90 to 100	2 to 3	8 to 12[a]	99	0.08 to 0.10	-------------
Etodolac (LODINE)	80 to 90	1 to 2	7 to 8	99	-------------	-------------
Fenoprofen Calcium (NALFON)	85 to 90	1 to 2	3	99	0.08 to 0.10	25 to 50
Flurbiprofen (ANSAID)	90 to 100	1 to 2	3 to 9	99	-------------	10 to 20
Ibuprofen (ADVIL, MOTRIN, NUPRIN, etc.)	80 to 90	0.5 to 1.5	2	95 to 99	0.15 to 0.17	-------------
Indomethacin (INDOCIN)	95 to 98	2	2 to 3	90	0.25 to 0.30	0.3 to 1.0
Ketorolac Tromethamine (TORADOL)	99 to 100	0.5 to 0.6	4 to 6	99	0.15 to 0.33	-------------
Meclofenamate Sodium (MECLOMEN)	-------------	0.5 to 1	2	99	-------------	-------------
Mefenamic Acid (PONSTEL)	-------------	2 to 4	2	99	-------------	-------------
Nabumetone (RELAFEN)	80 to 100	3	24	99	0.7	-------------
Naproxen (NAPROSYN)	95 to 100	2 to 4	13 to 15	99	0.15 to 0.17	25 to 50
Naproxen Sodium (ANAPROX)	95 to 100	2 to 4	13 to 15	99	0.15 to 0.17	25 to 50
Oxaprozin (DAYPRO)	90 to 100	3 to 5	50	99	-------------	-------------
Phenylbutazone	80 to 100	1 to 3	60 100	98	0.09 to 0.10	50 to 150
Piroxicam (FELDENE)	90 to 100	3 to 5	30 to 80	99	0.12 to 0.14	1.5 to 2
Sulindac (CLINORIL)	85 to 95	2	7 to 18	90 to 95	-------------	-------------
Tolmetin Sodium (TOLECTIN)	90 to 100	0.5 to 1	1 to 2	99	0.09 to 0.12	-------------

[a] The elimination kinetics of salicylates are complex since some of the enzymes involved in the biotransformation of salicylates are saturable at therapeutic plasma concentrations. Therefore, the elimination half-life increases with dose, e.g., with salicylic acid: at 325 to 650 mg (administered as aspirin) the elimination half-life is 2 - 3 hours; at 1000 mg, it is 5 - 8 hours; and at 2000 mg, it is 8 - 16 hours.

[b] ------------- indicates that no data are available.

TABLE H. SELECTED INDIVIDUAL NON-OPIOID ANALGESIC PREPARATIONS

GENERIC NAME	TRADE NAME	DOSAGE FORMS	COMMON ADULT DOSAGE	COMMON PEDIATRIC DOSAGE
Acetaminophen	ASPIRIN FREE ANACIN	**Cplt, Tab & Gelcplt**: 500 mg	**Pain or Fever**: 1000 mg tid or qid po.	Not recommended for use in children under 12.
	BAYER SELECT HEADACHE	**Cplt**: 500 mg	**Pain or Fever**: 1000 mg tid or qid po.	Not recommended for use in children under 12.
	FEVERALL	**Rectal Suppos**: 120 mg		**Pain or Fever (3-6 yrs)**: Insert 1 rectally q 4 - 6 h.
		Rectal Suppos: 325 mg	**Pain or Fever**: Insert 2 rectally q 4 - 6 h.	**6-12 yrs**: Insert 1 rectally q 4 to 6 h.
	FEVERALL SPRINKLE CAPS - Children's Strength	**Cpsl**: 80 mg		**Pain or Fever**: Dosage based on age and weight and should not exceed 5 doses in 24 h. Repeat doses below q 4 h po- **4-23 mos (12-23 lbs)**: 80 mg. **2-3 yrs (24-35 lbs)**: 160 mg. **4-5 yrs (36-47 lbs)**: 240 mg. **6-8 yrs (48-59 lbs)**: 320 mg. **9-10 yrs (60-71 lbs)**: 400 mg. **11 yrs (72-95 lbs)**: 480 mg.
	FEVERALL SPRINKLE CAPS - Junior Strength	**Cpsl**: 160 mg		**Pain or Fever**: Dosage based on age and weight and should not exceed 5 doses in 24 h. Repeat doses below q 4 h po- **2-5 yrs (24-47 lbs)**: 160 mg. **6-10 yrs (48-71 lbs)**: 320 mg. **11 yrs (71-95 lbs)**: 480 mg. **12-14 yrs (95+ lbs)**: 640 mg.

LIQUIPRIN	**Solution (Drops)**: 80 mg per 1.66 mL		**Pain or Fever**: Dosage based on age and weight and should not exceed 5 doses in 24 h. Repeat doses below q 4 h po- **Under 3 mos (under 12 lbs)**: 40 mg. **4-11 mos (12-17 lbs)**: 80 mg. **12-23 mos (18-23 lbs)**: 120 mg. **2-3 yrs (24-35 lbs)**: 160 mg. **4-5 yrs (36-47 lbs)**: 240 mg.
PANADOL, CHILDREN'S	**Solution (Drops)**: 80 mg per 0.8 mL **Chewable Tab**: 80 mg **Liquid**: 160 mg/5 mL		**Pain or Fever**: Dosage based on age and weight and should not exceed 5 doses in 24 h. Repeat doses below q 4 h po- **Under 4 mos (6-11 lbs)**: 40 mg. **4-11 mos (12-17 lbs)**: 80 mg. **12-23 mos (18-23 lbs)**: 120 mg. **2-3 yrs (24-35 lbs)**: 160 mg. **4-5 yrs (36-47 lbs)**: 240 mg. **6-8 yrs (48-59 lbs)**: 320 mg. **9-10 yrs (60-71 lbs)**: 400 mg. **11-12 yrs (72-95 lbs)**: 480 mg.
PANADOL, JUNIOR STRENGTH	**Cplt**: 160 mg	**Pain or Fever**: 640 mg q 4 h po.	**Pain or Fever**: Dosage based on age and weight and should not exceed 5 doses in 24 h. Repeat doses below q 4 h po- **2-3 yrs (24-35 lbs)**: 160 mg. **4-5 yrs (36-47 lbs)**: 240 mg. **6-8 yrs (48-59 lbs)**: 320 mg. **9-10 yrs (60-71 lbs)**: 400 mg. **11-12 yrs (72-95 lbs)**: 480 mg.

GENERIC NAME	TRADE NAME	DOSAGE FORMS	COMMON ADULT DOSAGE	COMMON PEDIATRIC DOSAGE
Acetaminophen [continued]	PANADOL, MAXIMUM STRENGTH	**Cplt & Tab**: 500 mg	**Pain or Fever**: 1000 mg q 4 h po.	
	ST. JOSEPH ASPIRIN-FREE FOR CHILDREN	**Cplt**: 160 mg	**Pain or Fever**: 640 mg q 4 h po.	**Pain or Fever**: Dosage based on age and weight and should not exceed 5 doses in 24 h. Repeat doses below q 4 h po- **12-23 mos (22-26 lbs)**: 120 mg. **2-3 yrs (27-35 lbs)**: 160 mg. **4-5 yrs (36-45 lbs)**: 240 mg. **6-8 yrs (46-65 lbs)**: 320 mg. **9-10 yrs (66-76 lbs)**: 400 mg. **11 yrs (77-83 lbs)**: 480 mg.
	TEMPRA 1 TEMPRA 2 TEMPRA 3	**Solution (Drops)**: 80 mg per 0.8 mL **Syrup**: 160 mg/5 mL **Chewable Tab**: 80 mg **(Regular Strength)**, 160 mg **(Double Strength)**	**Pain or Fever**: 640 mg q 4 h po.	**Pain or Fever**: Dosage based on age and weight and should not exceed 5 doses in 24 h. Repeat doses below q 4 h po- **Under 4 mos (under 12 lbs)**: 40 mg. **4-11 mos (12-17 lbs)**: 80 mg. **12-23 mos (18-23 lbs)**: 120 mg. **2-3 yrs (24-35 lbs)**: 160 mg. **4-5 yrs (36-47 lbs)**: 240 mg. **6-8 yrs (48-59 lbs)**: 320 mg. **9-10 yrs (60-71 lbs)**: 400 mg. **11 yrs (72-95 lbs)**: 480 mg.

	TYLENOL, CHILDREN'S	**Solution (Drops)**: 80 mg per 0.8 mL **Chewable Tab**: 80 mg **Elixir**: 160 mg/5 mL		**Pain or Fever**: Dosage based on age and weight and should not exceed 5 doses in 24 h. Repeat doses below q 4 h po- **Under 3 mos (under 11 lbs)**: 40 mg. **4-11 mos (12-17 lbs)**: 80 mg. **12-23 mos (18-23 lbs)**: 120 mg. **2-3 yrs (24-35 lbs)**: 160 mg. **4-5 yrs (36-47 lbs)**: 240 mg. **6-8 yrs (48-59 lbs)**: 320 mg. **9-10 yrs (60-71 lbs)**: 400 mg. **11-12 yrs (72+ lbs)**: 480 mg.
	JUNIOR STRENGTH TYLENOL	**Cplt & Chewable Tab**: 160 mg	**Pain or Fever**: 640 mg q 4 h po.	**Pain or Fever**: Dosage based on age and weight and should not exceed 5 doses in 24 h. Repeat doses below q 4 h po- **6-8 yrs (48-59 lbs)**: 320 mg. **9-10 yrs (60-71 lbs)**: 400 mg. **11 yrs (72-95 lbs)**: 480 mg.
	TYLENOL, REGULAR STRENGTH	**Cplt & Tab**: 325 mg	**Pain or Fever**: 325 - 650 mg tid or qid po.	**Pain or Fever (6-12 yrs)**: 160 to 325 mg tid or qid po.
	TYLENOL, EXTRA-STRENGTH	**Cplt, Tab & Gelcap**: 500 mg **Liquid (per 15 mL)**: 500 mg (7% alcohol)	**Pain or Fever**: 1000 mg tid or qid po. **Pain or Fever**: 30 mL (1000 mg) q 4 - 6 h po.	Not recommended for use in children under 12.
Aspirin,[1] Plain	BAYER ASPIRIN, CHILDREN'S	**Chewable Tab**: 81 mg	**Pain or Fever**: 650 mg q 4 h po.	**Pain or Fever**: Dosage based on age and weight. Repeat doses below q 4 h po- **2-4 yrs (32-35 lbs)**: 162 mg. **4-6 yrs (36-45 yrs)**: 243 mg. **6-9 yrs (46-65 lbs)**: 324 mg. **9-11 yrs (66-76 yrs)**: 405 mg. **11-12 yrs (77-83 lbs)**: 486 mg.

GENERIC NAME	TRADE NAME	DOSAGE FORMS	COMMON ADULT DOSAGE	COMMON PEDIATRIC DOSAGE
Aspirin,[1] Plain [continued]	BAYER ASPIRIN	**Cplt & Tab**: 325 mg	**Pain or Fever**: 325 - 650 mg q 4 h po.	Not recommended for use in children under 12.
	BAYER ASPIRIN, MAXIMUM	**Cplt & Tab**: 500 mg	**Pain or Fever**: 500 - 1000 mg q 4 h po.	Not recommended for use in children under 12.
	BAYER ASPIRIN, 8-HOUR	**Timed-Release Tab**: 650 mg	**Pain**: 650 mg q 8 h po.	Not recommended for use in children under 12.
	BAYER ENTERIC ASPIRIN - Adult Low Strength	**Enteric-Coated Tab**: 81 mg	**Pain**: 325 - 650 mg q 4 h po.	Not recommended for use in children under 12.
	BAYER ENTERIC ASPIRIN - Adult Reg. Strength	**Enteric-Coated Cplt**: 325 mg	**Pain**: 325 - 650 mg q 4 h po.	Not recommended for use in children under 12.
	ECOTRIN	**Enteric-Coated Tab & Cplt**: 325 mg	**Pain**: 325 - 650 mg q 4 h po.	Not recommended for use in children under 12.
	NORWICH ASPIRIN - Regular Strength	**Tab**: 325 mg	**Pain or Fever**: 325 - 650 mg q 4 h po.	**Pain or Fever (3-6 yrs)**: 160 to 325 mg q 3 - 4 h po. **6-12 yrs**: 325 mg q 3 - 4 h po.
	NORWICH ASPIRIN - Maximum Strength	**Tab**: 500 mg	**Pain or Fever**: 500 mg q 3 h po or 1000 mg q 6 h po.	Not recommended for use in children under 12.
	NORWICH ENTERIC SAFETY COATED ASPIRIN	**Enteric-Coated Tab**: 325, 500 mg	**Pain**: 500 mg q 6 h po or 650 mg q 4 h po.	Not recommended for use in children under 12.
	ST. JOSEPH ADULT CHEWABLE ASPIRIN	**Chewable Cplt**: 81 mg	**Pain or Fever**: 325 - 650 mg q 4 h po.	Not recommended for use in children under 12.

Aspirin,[1] Buffered	ALKA-SELTZER EFFERVESCENT ANTACID & PAIN RELIEVER	**Effervescent Tab**: 325 mg buffered with sodium bicarbonate (1916 mg), citric acid (1000 mg)	**Pain**: 650 mg mixed with 6 fl. oz. of water and allow to dissolve. Drink solution q 4 h.	Not recommended for use in children under 12.
	ALKA-SELTZER, FLAVORED EFFERVESCENT ANTACID & PAIN RELIEVER	**Effervescent Tab**: 325 mg buffered with sodium bicarbonate (1710 mg), citric acid (1220 mg)	**Pain**: 650 mg mixed with 6 fl. oz. of water and allow to dissolve. Drink solution q 4 h.	Not recommended for use in children under 12.
	ALKA-SELTZER EXTRA STRENGTH ANTACID & PAIN RELIEVER	**Effervescent Tab**: 500 mg buffered with sodium bicarbonate (1985 mg), citric acid (1000 mg)	**Pain**: 1000 mg mixed with 6 fl. oz. of water and allow to dissolve. Drink solution q 4 h.	Not recommended for use in children under 12.
	ARTHRITIS PAIN FORMULA	**Cplt**: 500 mg buffered with aluminum hydroxide (27 mg), magnesium hydroxide (100 mg)	**Pain or Fever**: 1000 mg tid or qid po.	Not recommended for use in children under 12.
	ASCRIPTIN	**Tab**: 325 mg buffered with aluminum hydroxide gel, magnesium hydroxide, calcium carbonate	**Pain or Fever**: 650 - 975 mg qid po.	Not recommended for use in children under 12.
	ASCRIPTIN A/D	**Cplt**: 325 mg buffered with aluminum hydroxide gel, magnesium hydroxide, calcium carbonate	**Pain**: 650 - 975 mg qid po.	Not recommended for use in children under 12.
	ASCRIPTIN EXTRA STRENGTH	**Cplt**: 500 mg buffered with aluminum hydroxide gel (80 mg), magnesium hydroxide (80 mg), calcium carbonate	**Pain**: 1000 mg tid - qid po.	Not recommended for use in children under 12.
	BAYER PLUS	**Cplt**: 325 mg buffered with calcium carbonate, magnesium oxide, magnesium carbonate	**Pain or Fever**: 325 - 650 mg q 4 h po.	Not recommended for use in children under 12.

GENERIC NAME	TRADE NAME	DOSAGE FORMS	COMMON ADULT DOSAGE	COMMON PEDIATRIC DOSAGE
Aspirin,[1] Buffered [continued]	BAYER PLUS, EXTRA STRENGTH	**Cplt**: 500 mg buffered with calcium carbonate, magnesium oxide, magnesium carbonate	**Pain or Fever**: 500 - 1000 mg q 4 h po.	Not recommended for use in children under 12.
	BUFFERIN	**Cplt & Tab**: 325 mg buffered with calcium carbonate, magnesium oxide, magnesium carbonate	**Pain or Fever**: 1000 mg q 4 h po.	Not recommended for use in children under 12.
	BUFFERIN, ARTHRITIS STRENGTH	**Cplt**: 500 mg buffered with calcium carbonate, magnesium oxide, magnesium carbonate	**Pain**: 1000 mg q 6 h po.	Not recommended for use in children under 12.
	BUFFERIN, EXTRA STRENGTH	**Tab**: 500 mg buffered with calcium carbonate, magnesium oxide, magnesium carbonate	**Pain**: 1000 mg q 6 h po.	Not recommended for use in children under 12.
	CAMA ARTHRITIS PAIN RELIEVER	**Tab**: 500 mg buffered with aluminum hydroxide (150 mg), magnesium oxide (150 mg)	**Pain**: 1000 mg q 6 h po.	Not recommended for use in children under 12.
Choline Salicylate	ARTHROPAN	**Oral Liquid**: 870 mg/5 mL	**Arthritic Pain**: 870 mg q 3 - 4 h po.	Not recommended for use in children under 12.
Diclofenac Sodium	VOLTAREN	**Enteric-Coated Tab**: 25, 50, 75 mg	**Arthritis**: 50 mg tid - qid po or 75 mg bid po.	Not recommended for use in children.
Diflunisal	DOLOBID	**Tab**: 250, 500 mg	**Pain**: 1000 mg, followed by 500 mg q 8 to 12 h po or 500 mg, followed by 250 mg q 8 - 12 h po. **Arthritis**: 250 - 500 mg bid po.	Not recommended for use in children under 12.

Etodolac	LODINE	**Cpsl**: 200, 300 mg	**Pain**: 200 - 400 mg q 6 - 8 h po. **Arthritis**: 800 - 1200 mg/day in divided doses po, followed by dosage adjustments with the range of 600 - 1200 mg/day in divided doses (i.e., 400 mg bid or tid; 300 mg bid - qid; or 200 mg tid or qid).	Not recommended for use in children.
Fenoprofen Calcium	NALFON 200	**Cpsl**: 200 mg (equivalent to fenoprofen base)	**Pain**: 200 mg q 4 - 6 h po, prn.	Not recommended for use in children.
	NALFON	**Cpsl**: 300 mg **Tab**: 600 mg	**Arthritis**: 300 - 600 mg tid to qid po.	
Flurbiprofen	ANSAID	**Tab**: 50, 100 mg	**Arthritis**: 50 mg qid po or 100 mg tid po.	Not recommended for use in children under 12.
Ibuprofen	ADVIL, MEDIPREN, MOTRIN IB, NUPRIN	**Cplt & Tab**: 200 mg	**Pain or Fever**: 200 - 400 mg q 4 - 6 h po, prn pain.	Not recommended for use in children under 12.
	BAYER SELECT IBUPROFEN, HALTRAN	**Tab**: 200 mg	**Pain or Fever**: 200 - 400 mg q 4 - 6 h po, prn pain.	Not recommended for use in children under 12.
	MOTRIN	**Tab**: 300, 400, 600, 800 mg	**Pain**: 400 mg q 4 - 6 h po, prn pain. **Arthritis**: 300 mg qid po or 600 - 800 mg tid to qid po.	Not recommended for use in children under 12.
	CHILDREN'S ADVIL, CHILDREN'S MOTRIN	**Susp**: 100 mg/5 mL	**Pain**: 400 mg q 4 - 6 h po, prn pain.	**Pain or Fever (over 6 months)**: 5 mg/kg if the baseline body temperature is 102.5 ^{O}F or below or 10 mg/kg if the baseline body temperature is over 102.5 ^{O}F. The duration of fever reduction is generally 6 - 8 h and longer with the higher dose.

GENERIC NAME	TRADE NAME	DOSAGE FORMS	COMMON ADULT DOSAGE	COMMON PEDIATRIC DOSAGE
Indomethacin	INDOCIN	**Cpsl**: 25, 50 mg	**Arthritis**: 25 - 50 mg bid - tid po. **Acute Painful Shoulder**: 25 - 50 mg tid po. **Acute Gout**: 50 mg tid po until the pain is tolerable.	Not recommended for use in children under 14.
		Oral Suspension: 25 mg/5 mL	**Arthritis**: 5 - 10 mL bid - tid po. **Acute Painful Shoulder**: 5 - 10 mL tid po. **Acute Gout**: 10 mL tid po until the pain is tolerable.	Not recommended for use in children under 14.
		Rectal Suppos: 50 mg	**Arthritis**: 50 mg rectally hs.	Not recommended for use in children under 14.
	INDOCIN SR	**Cpsl**: 75 mg	**Arthritis**: 75 mg once daily po.	Not recommended for use in children under 14.
Ketoprofen	ORUDIS	**Cpsl**: 25, 50, 75 mg	**Pain**: 25 - 50 mg q 6 - 8 h po, prn pain. **Arthritis**: 50 - 75 mg tid - qid po.	Not recommended for use in children.
Ketorolac Tromethamine	TORADOL	**Tab**: 10 mg	**Pain**: 10 mg q 4 - 6 h po for limited duration (average duration - 5 to 14 days).	Not recommended for use in children.
		Inj (per mL): 15, 30 mg	**Pain**: 30 - 60 mg IM, as a loading dose, followed by half of the loading dose (15 - 30 mg) q 6 h for up to 5 days. The lower end of the dosage range is recommended for patients under 50 kg (110 lbs), for patients over 65 years of age, and those with reduced renal function.	Not recommended for use in children.
Magnesium Salicylate	DOAN'S, REGULAR STRENGTH	**Cplt**: 325 mg	**Pain**: 650 mg q 4 h po, prn.	Not recommended for use in children.

	DOAN'S, EXTRA STRENGTH	**Cplt**: 500 mg	**Pain**: 1000 mg tid or qid po.	Not recommended for use in children.
	MAGAN	**Tab**: 545 mg (equivalent to 500 mg of salicylate base)	**Pain**: 545 mg q 4 h po or 1090 mg tid po.	Not recommended for use in children.
Meclofenamate Sodium	MECLOMEN	**Cpsl**: 50, 100 mg (equivalent to meclofenamic acid)	**Pain**: 50 mg q 4 - 6 h po. **Arthritis**: 50 - 100 mg tid - qid po.	Not recommended for use in children under 14.
Mefenamic Acid	PONSTEL	**Cpsl**: 250 mg	**Pain**: 500 mg initially, then 250 mg q 6 h po.	Not recommended for use in children under 14.
Nabumetone	RELAFEN	**Tab**: 500, 750 mg	**Arthritis**: Initially 1000 mg po as a single dose with or without food. Dosage may be increased to 1500 - 2000 mg/day as a single dose or in 2 divided doses.	
Naproxen	NAPROSYN	**Suspension**: 125 mg/5 mL	**Pain**: 20 mL (500 mg) initially, then 10 mL (250 mg) q 6 - 8 h po. **Acute Gout**: 30 mL (750 mg), followed by 10 mL (250 mg) 8 h po until the attack subsides. **Arthritis**: 10 - 20 mL (250 - 500 mg) bid po (morning and evening).	**Pain**: not recommended for use in children. **Juvenile Arthritis (Over 2 yrs)**: 2.5 - 5 mg/kg bid po with the total daily dose not exceeding 15 mg/kg/day.
		Tab: 250, 375, 500 mg	**Pain**: 500 mg initially, then 250 mg q 6 - 8 h po. **Acute Gout**: 750 mg followed by 250 mg q 8 h po until the attack subsides. **Arthritis**: 250 - 500 mg bid po (morning and evening).	**Pain**: not recommended for use in children. **Juvenile Arthritis (Over 2 yrs)**: same as above.
Naproxen Sodium	ANAPROX	**Tab**: 275 mg (equivalent to 250 mg of naproxen base)	**Pain**: 550 mg initially, then 275 mg q 6 - 8 h po. **Acute Gout**: 825 mg followed by 275 mg q 8 h po until the attack subsides.	**Pain**: not recommended for use in children. **Juvenile Arthritis (Over 2 yrs)**: 10 mg/kg/day po [NAPROSYN Suspension recommended].
	ANAPROX DS	**Tab**: 550 mg (equivalent to 500 mg of naproxen base)	**Arthritis**: 275 - 550 mg bid po (morning and evening).	

GENERIC NAME	TRADE NAME	DOSAGE FORMS	COMMON ADULT DOSAGE	COMMON PEDIATRIC DOSAGE
Oxaprozin	DAYPRO	**Tab**: 600 mg	**Rheumatoid arthritis**: 1200 mg once daily po. **Osteoarthritis**: 600 - 1200 mg once daily po.	Not recommended for use in children.
Oxyphenbutazone		**Tab**: 100 mg	**Acute Gout**: 400 mg followed by 100 mg q 4 h po for no more than 7 days. **Arthritis**: 100 mg qid po.	Not recommended for use in children under 14.
Phenylbutazone		**Cpsl & Tab**: 100 mg	**Acute Gout**: 400 mg followed by 100 mg q 4 h po for no more than 7 days. **Arthritis**: 100 mg qid po.	Not recommended for use in children under 14.
Piroxicam	FELDENE	**Cpsl**: 10, 20 mg	**Arthritis**: 20 mg once daily po.	Not recommended for use in children.
Salsalate	DISALCID	**Cpsl**: 500 mg	**Arthritis**: 1500 mg bid po or 1000 mg tid po.	Not recommended for use in children.
	DISALCID, SALFLEX	**Tab**: 500, 750 mg	**Arthritis**: 1500 mg bid po or 1000 mg tid po	Not recommended for use in children.
Sodium Salicylate		**Enteric-Coated Tab**: 325, 650 mg	**Pain**: 325 - 650 mg q 4 h po.	Not recommended for use in children.
Sulindac	CLINORIL	**Tab**: 150, 200 mg	**Acute Painful Shoulder and Acute Gout**: 200 mg bid po. **Arthritis**: 150 mg bid po.	Not recommended for use in children.
Tolmetin Sodium	TOLECTIN 200	**Tab**: 200 mg (equivalent to tolmetin base)	**Arthritis**: 400 mg tid po.	**Juvenile Arthritis (over 2 yrs)**: 20 mg/kg/day in divided doses (tid or qid) po.
	TOLECTIN DS	**Cpsl**: 400 mg (equivalent to tolmetin base)	**Arthritis**: 400 mg tid po.	
	TOLECTIN 600	**Tab**: 600 mg (equivalent to tolmetin base)	**Arthritis**: 600 mg bid - tid po.	

1 Children and teenagers should not use aspirin for chicken pox or flu symptoms before a doctor is consulted about Reye Syndrome, a rare but serious illness.

TABLE I. SELECTED COMBINATION NON-OPIOID ANALGESIC PREPARATIONS

TRADE NAME	DOSAGE FORMS	COMMON ADULT DOSAGE	COMMON PEDIATRIC DOSAGE
ANACIN	**Cplt & Tab**: aspirin (400 mg), caffeine (32 mg)	**Pain or Fever**: 2 cplt (or tab) q 4 h po.	Not recommended for use in children under 6. **Pain or Fever (6-12 yrs)**: 1 cplt (or tab) q 4 h po.
ANACIN, MAXIMUM STRENGTH	**Tab**: aspirin (500 mg), caffeine (32 mg)	**Pain or Fever**: 2 tab tid - qid po.	Not recommended for use in children under 12.
ARTHRITIS STRENGTH BC POWDER	**Powder (per packet)**: aspirin (742 mg), salicylamide (222 mg), caffeine (36 mg)	**Pain or Fever**: Stir powder into a glass of water or other liquid. Drink q 3 - 4 h, up to 4 powders per 24 h.	Not recommended for use in children under 12.
BC POWDER	**Powder (per packet)**: aspirin (650 mg), salicylamide (195 mg), caffeine (32 mg)	**Pain or Fever**: Stir powder into a glass of water or other liquid. Drink q 3 - 4 h, up to qid.	Not recommended for use in children under 12.
DOAN'S P.M.	**Cplt**: magnesium salicylate (500 mg), diphenhydramine HCl (25 mg)	**Pain**: 2 cplt po hs prn.	Not recommended for use in children under 12.
EQUAGESIC (C-IV)	**Tab**: aspirin (325 mg), meprobamate (200 mg)	**Pain**: 1 - 2 tab tid - qid po.	Not recommended for use in children under 12.
EXCEDRIN	**Cplt & Tab**: acetaminophen (250 mg), aspirin (250 mg), caffeine (65 mg)	**Pain or Fever**: 2 cplt (or tab) q 4 h po.	Not recommended for use in children under 12.
EXCEDRIN, ASPIRIN FREE	**Cplt**: acetaminophen (500 mg), caffeine (65 mg)	**Pain or Fever**: 2 cplt q 6 h po while symptoms persist.	Not recommended for use in children under 12.
FIORICET	**Tab**: acetaminophen (325 mg), caffeine (40 mg), butalbital (50 mg)	**Tension Headache**: 1 - 2 tab q 4 h po, prn.	Not recommended for use in children under 12.

TRADE NAME	DOSAGE FORMS	COMMON ADULT DOSAGE	COMMON PEDIATRIC DOSAGE
FIORINAL (C-III)	**Cpsl & Tab**: aspirin (325 mg), caffeine (40 mg), butalbital (50 mg)	**Tension Headache**: 1 - 2 cpsl (or tab) q 4 h po, prn.	Not recommended for use in children under 12.
MICRAININ (C-IV)	**Tab**: aspirin (325 mg), meprobamate (200 mg)	**Pain**: 1 - 2 tab tid - qid po.	Not recommended for use in children under 12.
MOBIGESIC	**Tab**: magnesium salicylate (325 mg), phenyltoloxamine citrate (30 mg)	**Pain**: 1 - 2 tab q 4 h po, up to 10 tab daily.	**Pain (6-12 yrs)**: 1 tab q 4 h po, up to 5 tab daily.
MOMENTUM	**Cplt**: aspirin (500 mg), phenyltoloxamine citrate (15 mg)	**Pain**: 2 cplt po on arising, then 2 cplt prn at lunch, dinner, and bedtime.	Not recommended for use in children.
NORGESIC	**Tab**: aspirin (385 mg), caffeine (30 mg), orphenadrine citrate (25 mg)	**Musculoskeletal Pain**: 1 - 2 tab tid to qid po.	Not recommended for use in children.
NORGESIC FORTE	Tab: aspirin (770 mg), caffeine (60 mg), orphenadrine citrate (50 mg)	**Musculoskeletal Pain**: 1/2 - 1 tab tid to qid po.	Not recommended for use in children.
P-A-C	**Tab**: aspirin (400 mg), anhydrous caffeine (32 mg)	**Pain or Fever**: 1 - 2 tab q 4 h po.	Not recommended for use in children under 12.
PERCOGESIC	**Tab**: acetaminophen (325 mg), phenyltoloxamine citrate (30 mg)	**Pain or Fever**: 1 - 2 tab q 4 h po, up to 8 tab per day.	**Pain or Fever (6-12 yrs)**: 1 tab q 4 h po, up to 4 tab per day.
PHRENILIN	**Tab**: acetaminophen (325 mg), butalbital (50 mg)	**Tension Headache**: 1 - 2 tab q 4 h po, prn.	Not recommended for use in children under 12.
PHRENILIN FORTE	**Cpsl**: acetaminophen (650 mg), butalbital (50 mg)	**Tension Headache**: 1 cpsl q 4 h po, prn.	Not recommended for use in children under 12.
ROBAXISAL	**Tab**: aspirin (325 mg), methocarbamol (400 mg)	**Musculoskeletal Pain**: 2 tab qid po.	Not recommended for use in children under 12.
SOMA COMPOUND	**Tab**: aspirin (325 mg), carisoprodol (200 mg)	**Musculoskeletal Pain**: 1 - 2 tab qid po.	Not recommended for use in children under 12.

TRILISATE	**Oral Liquid (per 5 mL)**: choline magnesium salicylate (500 mg as: choline salicylate (293 mg) and magnesium salicylate (362 mg) **Tab**: choline magnesium salicylate (500 mg as: choline salicylate (293 mg) and magnesium salicylate (362 mg)) **Tab**: choline magnesium salicylate (750 mg as: choline salicylate (440 mg) and magnesium salicylate (544 mg)) **Tab**: choline magnesium salicylate (1000 mg as: choline salicylate (587 mg) and magnesium salicylate (725 mg))	**Pain or Fever**: 2000 - 3000 mg daily po in divided doses (bid). **Arthritis**: 3000 mg once daily po hs or 1500 mg bid po.	**Pain or Fever**: Total daily doses shown below should be given in divided doses (bid) po. **12-13 kg**: 500 mg. **14-17 kg**: 750 mg. **18-22 kg**: 1000 mg. **23-27 kg**: 1250 mg. **28-32 kg**: 1500 mg. **33-37 kg**: 1750 mg. **Over 37 kg**: 2250 mg.
TYLENOL, EXTRA STRENGTH HEADACHE PLUS	**Cplt**: acetaminophen (500 mg), calcium carbonate (250 mg)	**Pain**: 2 cplt q 6 h po.	Not recommended for use in children under 12.
VANQUISH	**Cplt**: acetaminophen (194 mg), aspirin (227 mg), caffeine (33 mg), dried aluminum hydroxide gel (25 mg), magnesium hydroxide (50 mg)	**Pain**: 2 cplt q 4 h po, prn.	Not recommended for use in children under 12.

(C-III): Schedule III, Controlled Substances Act
(C-IV): Schedule IV, Controlled Substances Act

TABLE J. SELECTED COMBINATION NON-OPIOID ANALGESIC PREPARATIONS CONTAINING SLEEP AIDS

TRADE NAME	DOSAGE FORMS	COMMON ADULT DOSAGE	COMMON PEDIATRIC DOSAGE
ANACIN P.M., ASPIRIN FREE	**Cplt**: acetaminophen (500 mg), diphenhydramine HCl (25 mg)	**Pain**: 2 cplt hs po, prn.	Not recommended for use in children under 12.
BAYER SELECT NIGHT TIME PAIN RELIEF	**Cplt**: acetaminophen (500 mg), diphenhydramine HCl (25 mg)	**Pain**: 2 cplt hs po prn.	Not recommended for use in children under 12.
BUFFERIN AF NITE-TIME	**Cplt**: acetaminophen (500 mg), diphenhydramine citrate (38 mg)	**Pain**: 2 cplt po hs prn.	Not recommended for use in children under 12.
EXCEDRIN P.M.	**Cplt & Tab**: acetaminophen (500 mg), diphenhydramine citrate (38 mg)	**Pain**: 2 cplt (or tab) po, hs.	Not recommended for use in children under 12.
	Liquid (per 30 mL): acetaminophen (1000 mg), diphenhydramine HCl (50 mg), alcohol (10%)	**Pain**: 30 mL po hs, prn.	Not recommended for use in children under 12.
MIDOL PM	**Cplt**: acetaminophen (500 mg), diphenhydramine HCl (25 mg)	**Pain**: 2 cplt po hs, prn.	Not recommended for use in children under 12.
SOMINEX PAIN RELIEF FORMULA	**Tab**: acetaminophen (500 mg), diphenhydramine HCl (25 mg)	**Pain**: 2 tab po, 30 minutes before bedtime.	Not recommended for use in children under 12.
TYLENOL PM, EXTRA STRENGTH	**Cplt, Tab & Gelcap**: acetaminophen (500 mg), diphenhydramine HCl (25 mg)	**Pain**: 2 cplt (or tab or gelcap) po, hs.	Not recommended for use in children under 12.
UNISOM WITH PAIN RELIEF	**Tab**: acetaminophen (650 mg), diphenhydramine HCl (50 mg)	**Pain**: 1 tab po 30 minutes before bedtime.	Not recommended for use in children under 12.

TABLE K. SELECTED COMBINATION OPIOID AND NON-OPIOID ANALGESIC PREPARATIONS

TRADE NAME	DOSAGE FORMS AND COMPOSITION	COMMON ADULT DOSAGE	COMMON PEDIATRIC DOSAGE
ANEXSIA 5/500	**Tab**: acetaminophen (500 mg), hydrocodone bitartrate (5 mg)	1 - 2 tab q 4 - 6 h po, prn pain.	Not recommended for use in children.
ANEXSIA 7.5/650	**Tab**: acetaminophen (650 mg), hydrocodone bitartrate (7.5 mg)	1 tab q 4 - 6 h po, prn pain.	Not recommended for use in children.
DARVOCET-N 50 (C-IV)	**Tab**: acetaminophen (325 mg), propoxyphene napsylate (50 mg)	1 - 2 tab q 4 h po, prn pain.	Not recommended for use in children.
DARVOCET-N 100 (C-IV)	**Tab**: acetaminophen (650 mg), propoxyphene napsylate (100 mg)	1 tab q 4 h po, prn pain.	Not recommended for use in children.
DARVON COMPOUND-65 (C-IV)	**Cpsl**: aspirin (389 mg), caffeine (32.4 mg), propoxyphene hydrochloride (65 mg)	1 cpsl q 4 h po, prn pain.	Not recommended for use in children.
EMPIRIN W/CODEINE NO. 3	**Tab**: aspirin (325 mg), codeine phosphate (30 mg)	1 - 2 tab q 4 h po, prn pain.	
EMPIRIN W/CODEINE NO. 4	**Tab**: aspirin (325 mg), codeine phosphate (60 mg)	1 tab q 4 h po, prn pain.	
FIORICET W/CODEINE	**Cpsl**: acetaminophen (325 mg), caffeine (40 mg), butalbital (50 mg), codeine phosphate (30 mg)	1 - 2 cpsl q 4 h po, prn pain.	Not recommended for use in children under 12.
FIORINAL W/CODEINE	**Cpsl**: aspirin (325 mg), caffeine (40 mg), butalbital (50 mg), codeine phosphate (30 mg)	1 - 2 cpsl q 4 h po, prn pain.	Not recommended for use in children under 12.
HYDROCET	**Cpsl**: acetaminophen (500 mg), hydrocodone bitartrate (5 mg)	1 - 2 cpsl q 4 - 6 h po, prn pain.	Not recommended for use in children.
LORTAB	**Liquid (per 5 mL)**: hydrocodone bitartrate (2.5 mg), acetaminophen (120 mg), alcohol (7%)	15 mL q 4 h po, prn pain.	Safety and effectiveness in children have not been established.

LORTAB 2.5/500	**Tab**: hydrocodone bitartrate (2.5 mg), acetaminophen (500 mg)	1 - 2 tab q 4 - 6 h po, prn pain.	Safety and effectiveness in children have not been established.
LORTAB 5/500	**Tab**: hydrocodone bitartrate (5 mg), acetaminophen (500 mg)	1 - 2 tab q 4 - 6 h po, prn pain.	Safety and effectiveness in children have not been established.
LORTAB 7.5/500	**Tab**: hydrocodone bitartrate (7.5 mg), acetaminophen (500 mg)	1 tab q 4 - 6 h po, prn pain.	Safety and effectiveness in children have not been established.
LORTAB ASA	**Tab**: hydrocodone bitartrate (5 mg), aspirin (500 mg)	1 - 2 tab q 4 - 6 h po, prn pain.	Safety and effectiveness in children have not been established.
PERCOCET (C-II)	**Tab**: acetaminophen (325 mg), oxycodone hydrochloride (5 mg)	1 tab q 6 h po, prn pain.	Not recommended for use in children.
PERCODAN (C-II)	**Tab**: aspirin (325 mg), oxycodone hydrochloride (5 mg)	1 tab q 6 h po, prn pain.	Not recommended for use in children.
PERCODAN-DEMI (C-II)	**Tab**: aspirin (325 mg), oxycodone hydrochloride (2.5 mg)	1 - 2 tab q 6 h po, prn pain.	Not recommended for use in children under 6. **6-12 yrs**: 1/4 tab q 6 h po. **Over 12 yrs**: 1/2 tab q 6 h po.
PHENAPHEN W/CODEINE NO. 2	**Cpsl**: acetaminophen (300 mg), codeine phosphate (15 mg)	1 - 2 cpsl q 4 h po, prn pain po.	**Over 3 yrs**: Based on codeine dose of 0.5 mg/kg up to q **4** h po.
PHENAPHEN W/CODEINE NO. 3	**Cpsl**: acetaminophen (300 mg), codeine phosphate (30 mg)	1 - 2 cpsl q 4 h prn pain po.	**Over 3 yrs**: Based on codeine dose of 0.5 mg/kg up to q **4** h po.
PHENAPHEN W/CODEINE NO. 4	**Cpsl**: acetaminophen (300 mg), codeine phosphate (60 mg)	1 cpsl q 4 h prn pain po.	**Over 3 yrs**: Based on codeine dose of 0.5 mg/kg up to q **4** h po.

TRADE NAME	DOSAGE FORMS AND COMPOSITION	COMMON ADULT DOSAGE	COMMON PEDIATRIC DOSAGE
PHENAPHEN-650 W/CODEINE	**Tab**: acetaminophen (650 mg), codeine phosphate (30 mg)	1 tab q 4 h prn pain po.	**Over 3 yrs**: Based on codeine dose of 0.5 mg/kg up to q 4 h po.
ROXICET (C-II)	**Tab**: acetaminophen (325 mg), oxycodone hydrochloride (5 mg) **Oral Solution (per 5 mL)**: acetaminophen (325 mg), oxycodone hydrochloride (5 mg), alcohol (0.4%)	1 tab q 6 h po, prn pain. 5 mL q 6 h po, prn pain.	Not recommended for use in children. Not recommended for use in children.
ROXICET 5/500 (C-II)	**Cplt**: acetaminophen (500 mg), oxycodone hydrochloride (5 mg)	1 cplt q 6 h po, prn pain.	Not recommended for use in children.
ROXIPRIN (C-II)	**Tab**: aspirin (325 mg), oxycodone hydrochloride (5 mg)	1 tab q 6 h po, prn pain.	Not recommended for use in children.
SYNALGOS-DC	**Cpsl**: aspirin (356.4 mg), caffeine (30 mg), dihydrocodeine bitartrate (16 mg)	2 cpsl q 4 h po, prn pain.	Not recommended for use in children under 12.
TALACEN (C-IV)	**Cplt**: acetaminophen (650 mg), pentazocine hydrochloride (25 mg)	1 cplt q 4 h po, prn pain.	Not recommended for use in children under 12.
TALWIN COMPOUND (C-IV)	**Cplt**: aspirin (325 mg), pentazocine hydrochloride (12.5 mg)	2 cplt tid to qid po.	Not recommended for use in children under 12.
TYLENOL W/CODEINE (C-V)	**Elixir (per 5 mL)**: acetaminophen (120 mg), codeine phosphate (12 mg), alcohol (7%)	15 mL q 4 h prn pain po.	Not recommended for use in children under 3. **3-6 yrs**: 5 mL tid to qid po. **7-12 yrs**: 10 mL tid to qid po.
TYLENOL W/CODEINE NO. 1	**Tab**: acetaminophen (300 mg), codeine phosphate (7.5 mg)	1 - 2 tab 4 h prn pain po.	**Over 3 yrs**: Based on codeine dose of 0.5 mg/kg up to q 4 h po.
TYLENOL W/CODEINE NO. 2	**Tab**: acetaminophen (300 mg), codeine phosphate (15 mg)	1 - 2 tab q 4 h prn pain po.	**Over 3 yrs**: Based on codeine dose of 0.5 mg/kg up to q 4 h po.

TYLENOL W/CODEINE NO. 3	**Tab**: acetaminophen (300 mg), codeine phosphate (30 mg)	1 - 2 tab q 4 h prn pain po.	**Over 3 yrs**: Based on codeine dose of 0.5 mg/kg up to q 4 h po.
TYLENOL W/CODEINE NO. 4	**Tab**: acetaminophen (300 mg), codeine phosphate (60 mg)	1 tab q 4 h prn pain po.	**Over 3 yrs**: Based on codeine dose of 0.5 mg/kg up to q 4 h po.
TYLOX (C-II)	**Cpsl**: acetaminophen (500 mg), oxycodone hydrochloride (5 mg)	1 cpsl q 6 h po, prn pain.	Not recommended for use in children.
VICODIN	**Tab**: acetaminophen (500 mg), hydrocodone bitartrate (5 mg)	1 - 2 tab q 4 - 6 h po, prn pain.	Not recommended for use in children.
VICODIN ES	**Tab**: acetaminophen (750 mg), hydrocodone bitartrate (7.5 mg)	1 tab q 4 - 6 h po, prn pain.	Not recommended for use in children.
WYGESIC (C-IV)	**Tab**: acetaminophen (650 mg), propoxyphene hydrochloride (65 mg)	1 tab q 4 h po, prn pain.	Not recommended for use in children.
ZYDONE	**Cpsl**: acetaminophen (500 mg), hydrocodone bitartrate (5 mg)	1 - 2 cpsl q 4 - 6 h po, prn pain.	Not recommended for use in children.

All of these products are classified as Schedule III (C-III) under the Controlled Substance Act unless otherwise noted.

(C-II): Schedule II, Controlled Substances Act
(C-IV): Schedule IV, Controlled Substances Act
(C-V): Schedule V, Controlled Substances Act

TABLE L. APPROACH TO CLINICAL PROBLEMS ASSOCIATED WITH NSAID USE

PROBLEM	RECOMMENDED THERAPY
Active peptic ulcer	Use a nonulcerogenic analgesic, e.g., acetaminophen, with or without an opioid analgesic.
History of peptic ulcer or gastrointestinal bleeding	Administer the NSAID with food, an antacid, sucralfate, or an H_2-receptor blocker (see Table Q); monitor clinical status closely.
Platelet abnormalities	Avoid NSAIDs.
Anticipated surgery	Discontinue NSAIDs (especially aspirin).
Concurrent warfarin therapy	Use ibuprofen, naproxen or tolmetin with caution; avoid phenylbutazone and salicylates.
Renal disease and low volume states	Do baseline urinalysis, electrolytes and creatinine; discontinue NSAID for weight gain, proteinuria or elevation in BUN, creatinine, or potassium.
Hypertension	Monitor blood pressure closely.
Geriatric patients	Watch closely for changes in mental status and discontinue NSAID for disorientation, irritability, depression, etc.

TABLE M. COMPARISON OF SELECTED CORTICOSTEROIDS

DRUG	EQUIVALENT DOSE (mg)[a]	RELATIVE ANTI-INFLAMMATORY POTENCY	RELATIVE MINERALOCORTICOID POTENCY
SHORT DURATION			
Cortisone	25.0	0.8	2.0
Hydrocortisone	20.0	1.0	2.0
INTERMEDIATE DURATION			
Prednisone	5.0	4.0	1.0
Prednisolone	5.0	4.0	1.0
Methylprednisolone	4.0	5.0	0.5
Triamcinolone	4.0	5.0	0
LONG DURATION			
Paramethasone	2.0	10.0	0
Dexamethasone	0.75	25.0	0
Betamethasone	0.6	30.0	0

[a] Based on oral administration.

TABLE N. SELECTED ANALGESIC ADJUVANTS

GENERIC NAME	TRADE NAME	CLASSIFICATION	THERAPEUTIC USES	DOSAGE FORMS	COMMON ADULT DOSE
Alprazolam (C-IV)	XANAX	Anxiolytic	Anxiety	**Tab**: 0.25, 0.5, 1, 2 mg	0.25 - 0.5 mg tid po.
Amitriptyline Hydrochloride	ELAVIL, ENDEP	Antidepressant	Potentiation of opioid analgesics[1]	**Tab**: 10, 25, 50, 75, 100, 150 mg	**Depression - Outpatients:** Initially, 25 mg tid po; may be increased to 50 mg tid po if necessary. The usual maintenance dose is 50 - 100 mg daily po. **Depression - Hospitalized Patients:** Initially, these patients may require up to 100 mg daily po; may be increased to 200 mg daily if necessary. The usual maintenance dose is 50 to 100 mg daily po. **Adolescent Patients:** 10 mg tid po, with 20 mg hs, may be acceptable.
	ELAVIL			**Inj**: 10 mg/mL	Initially, 20 - 30 mg qid IM. Amitriptyline tablets should replace the injection as soon as possible.
Baclofen	LIORESAL	Skeletal Muscle Relaxant	Muscle spasticity and rigidity	**Tab**: 10, 20 mg	5 mg tid po for 3 days; increase by 5 mg tid q 3 days (maximum 80 mg daily (20 mg qid)) until optimum effect is achieved.

Buspirone Hydrochloride	BUSPAR	Anxiolytic	Anxiety	**Tab**: 5, 10 mg	5 mg tid po. Dosage may be increased 5 mg daily at 2 to 3 day intervals. Maximum: 60 mg per day.
Caffeine	NODOZ VIVARIN	CNS Stimulant	Potentiation of non-opioid analgesics[1]	**Tab**: 100 mg **Tab**: 200 mg	100 - 200 mg q 4 h po. 200 mg q 4 h po.
Carbamazepine	TEGRETOL	Anticonvulsant	Pain associated with trigeminal neuralgia	**Susp**: 100 mg/5 mL **Chewable Tab**: 100 mg **Tab**: 200 mg	**Initial**: 2.5 mL (Susp.) qid po or 100 mg (Tab) bid po on the first day. This daily dose may be increased by up to 200 mg daily using increments of 2.5 mL (Susp.) qid or 100 mg (Tab.) q 12 h po. Max.: 1200 mg daily. **Maintenance**: Adjust to minimum effective levels; usually 400 to 800 mg daily po.
Carisoprodol	SOMA	Skeletal Muscle Relaxant	Musculo-skeletal pain	**Tab**: 350 mg	350 mg tid and hs po.
Chlorphenesin Carbamate	MAOLATE	Skeletal Muscle Relaxant	Musculo-skeletal pain	**Tab**: 400 mg	Initially, 800 mg tid po until the desired effect is obtained; then 400 mg qid po.
Chlorzoxazone	PARAFLEX PARAFON FORTE DSC	Skeletal Muscle Relaxant	Musculo-skeletal pain	**Cplt**: 250 mg **Cplt**: 500 mg	250 mg tid or qid po. 500 mg tid or qid po.
Cyclobenzaprine Hydrochloride	FLEXERIL	Skeletal Muscle Relaxant	Musculo-skeletal pain	**Tab**: 10 mg	10 mg tid po.

GENERIC NAME	TRADE NAME	CLASSIFICATION	THERAPEUTIC USES	DOSAGE FORMS	COMMON ADULT DOSE
Dantrolene Sodium	DANTRIUM	Skeletal Muscle Relaxant	Muscle spasticity	**Cpsl**: 25, 50, 100 mg	Begin with 25 mg once daily po; increase to 25 mg bid to qid and then by increments of 25 mg. Maximum po dose is 400 mg daily.
Desipramine Hydrochloride	NORPRAMIN	Antidepressant	Potentiation of opioid analgesics[1]	**Tab**: 10, 25, 50, 75, 100, 150 mg	**Depression**: 100 to 200 mg daily po in a single dose or in divided doses.
Dextroamphetamine Sulfate (C-II)	DEXEDRINE	CNS Stimulant	Potentiation of opioid analgesics[1]; reduction of sedation[1]	**Tab**: 5 mg	**Narcolepsy**: 5 to 60 mg daily po, in divided doses depending on the patient's response.
Diazepam (C-IV)	VALIUM	Anxiolytic, Skeletal Muscle Relaxant	Muscle spasticity	**Tab**: 2, 5, 10 mg **Inj**: 5 mg/mL	2 - 10 mg tid to qid po. 5 - 10 mg IM or IV. Repeat in 3 to 4 h prn.
	VALRELEASE			**Slow-Rel. Cpsl**: 15 mg	15 - 30 mg once daily po.
Fluphenazine Hydrochloride	PROLIXIN	Antipsychotic	Potentiation of opioid analgesics[1]	**Tab**: 1, 2.5, 5, 10 mg **Elixir**: 2.5 mg/5 mL (14% alcohol) **Conc Liquid**: 5 mg/mL (14% alcohol)	**Psychosis**: 2.5 - 10 mg po daily in divided doses at 6- to 8-hour intervals.
				Inj: 2.5 mg/mL	**Psychosis**: 1.25 - 10 mg IM daily in divided doses at 6- to 8-hour intervals.
Fluphenazine Decanoate	PROLIXIN DECANOATE	Antipsychotic	Potentiation of opioid analgesics[1]	**Inj**: 25 mg/mL	**Psychosis**: 12.5 - 25 mg IM or SC.

Fluphenazine Enanthate	PROLIXIN ENANTHATE	Antipsychotic	Potentiation of opioid analgesics[1]	**Inj**: 25 mg/mL	**Psychosis**: 25 mg IM or SC q 2 weeks.
Haloperidol	HALDOL	Antipsychotic	Potentiation of opioid analgesics[1]	**Tab**: 0.5, 1, 2, 5, 10, 20 mg	**Psychosis**: 0.5 - 5 mg bid to tid po.
Haloperidol Decanoate	HALDOL DECANOATE 50 HALDOL DECANOATE 100	Antipsychotic	Potentiation of opioid analgesics[1]	**Inj**: 70.5 mg/mL (50 mg/mL as the base) **Inj**: 141.0 mg/mL (100 mg/mL as the base)	**Psychosis**: Give once q 4 weeks by deep IM injection. For patients previously maintained on antipsychotics, the recommended initial dose is 10 to 15 times the previous daily dose in oral haloperidol equivalents. The initial dose should not exceed 100 mg.
Haloperidol Lactate	HALDOL	Antipsychotic	Potentiation of opioid analgesics[1]	**Liquid Conc**: 2 mg/mL **Inj**: 5 mg/mL	**Psychosis**: 0.5 - 5 mg bid to tid po. **Psychosis**: 2 - 5 mg q 4 to 8 h IM.
Hydroxyzine Hydrochloride	ATARAX	Anxiolytic, Antihistamine	Potentiation of opioid analgesics	**Tab**: 10, 25, 50, 100 mg **Syrup**: 10 mg/5 mL (0.5% alcohol)	Oral doses should be individualized. 10 to 50 mg qid po is commonly used.
	VISTARIL			**Inj**: 25, 50 mg/mL	50 - 100 mg IM.
Hydroxyzine Pamoate	VISTARIL	Anxiolytic, Antihistamine	Potentiation of opioid analgesics	**Cpsl**: 25, 50, 100 mg **Suspension**: 25 mg/5 mL	Oral doses should be individualized. 10 to 50 mg qid po is commonly used.

GENERIC NAME	TRADE NAME	CLASSIFICATION	THERAPEUTIC USES	DOSAGE FORMS	COMMON ADULT DOSE
Imipramine Hydrochloride	TOFRANIL	Antidepressant	Potentiation of opioid analgesics[1]	**Tab**: 10, 25, 50 mg	**Depression - Outpatients:** Initially, 75 mg/day po in divided doses, increased to 150 mg/day. **Depression - Hospitalized Patients**: Initially, 100 mg/day po in divided doses, gradually increased to 200 mg/day po as required.
			Potentiation of opioid analgesics[1]	**Inj**: 25 mg/2 mL	**Depression**: Up to 100 mg/day IM in divided doses.
Methocarbamol	ROBAXIN	Skeletal Muscle Relaxant	Musculo-skeletal pain	**Tab**: 500 mg	**Initial**: 500 mg qid po. **Maintenance**: 1000 mg qid po.
	ROBAXIN-750			**Tab**: 750 mg	**Initial**: 1500 mg qid po. **Maintenance**: 750 mg q 4 h po or 1500 mg tid po.
Nortiptyline Hydrochloride	AVENTYL	Antidepressant	Potentiation of opioid analgesics[1]	**Cpsl**: 10, 25, 50, 75 mg **Liquid**: 10 mg/5 mL (4% alcohol)	**Depression**: 25 mg tid or qid po; or, total daily dose may be given once daily po.
Orphenadrine Citrate	NORFLEX	Skeletal Muscle Relaxant	Musculo-skeletal pain	**Tab**: 100 mg **Inj**: 60 mg/2 mL	100 mg bid po, AM and PM. 60 mg q 12 h deep IM or IV.

Phenytoin	DILANTIN	Antiepileptic	Neurological pain, i.e., trigeminal neuralgia[1]	**Susp**: 125 mg/5 mL	**Epilepsy**: Initially, 125 mg tid po; adjust dosage prn.
				Chewable Tab: 50 mg	**Epilepsy**: Initially, 100 mg tid po; adjust dosage prn.
Phentoin Sodium	DILANTIN	Antiepileptic	Neurological pain, i.e., trigeminal neuralgia[1]	**Cpsl**: 100 mg	**Epilepsy**: Initially, 100 mg tid po; adjust dosage prn. For patients controlled at 100 mg tid, a single daily dose of 300 mg po may be given.

1 Not an official FDA approved indication. The dosages given are for the FDA approved indication listed are are only to be used as guidance. Please see publications in the REFERENCE section of the chapter on MANAGEMENT OF PAIN for dosages used for these drugs as Analgesic Adjuvants.

(C-II): Schedule II, Controlled Substances Act
(C-IV): Schedule IV, Controlled Substances Act

TABLE 0. INJECTABLE ANTIHISTAMINE PREPARATIONS

GENERIC NAME	TRADE NAME	DOSAGE FORMS	COMMON ADULT DOSAGE	COMMON PEDIATRIC DOSAGE
Brompheniramine Maleate		**Solution**: 10 mg/mL	10 mg (range 5 - 20 mg) bid IM, SC or IV; maximum dose is 40 mg per 24 hours.	Under 12 yrs: 0.5 mg/kg/day or 15 mg/m^2/day in 3 to 4 divided doses IM, SC or IV.
Chlorpheniramine Maleate		**Solution**: 10 mg/mL (for IM, SC or IV use) **Solution**: 100 mg/mL (only for IM or SC use)	**Allergic Reaction**: 10 - 20 mg as a single dose IM, SC or IV to a maximum of 40 mg per 24 hours. **Anaphylaxis**: 10 - 20 mg as a single dose.	
Diphenhydramine Hydrochloride	BENADRYL	**Solution (per mL)**: 10, 50 mg	10 - 50 mg per dose IV or deep IM; maximum daily dose of 400 mg	5 mg/kg/24 hours or 150 mg/m^2/24 hours divided into 4 doses IV or deep IM. Maximum daily dose is 300 mg.
Promethazine Hydrochloride	PHENERGAN	**Solution (per mL)**: 25, 50 mg	**Allergic Reactions**: 25 mg IM or IV; may repeat in 2 hours if necessary. **Sedation**: 25 - 50 mg IM. **Pre- & Postoperative**: 25 to 50 mg IM or IV. **Nausea & Vomiting**: 12.5 to 25 mg q 4 h IM or IV. **Obstetrics**: 50 mg in the early stages of labor IM or IV; maximum dose is 100 mg/24 hours.	**Under 12 yrs**: Should not exceed half of the suggested adult dose. As an adjunct to premedication: 0.5 mg/lb IM or IV with an equal dose of opioid.

TABLE P. SELECTED LAXATIVES AND STOOL SOFTENERS

TRADE NAME	DOSAGE FORMS and ACTIVE INGREDIENTS	COMMON DOSAGES and ADMINISTRATION
AGORAL	**Liquid Emulsion (per 15 mL):** mineral oil (4.2 g), phenolphthalein (200 mg) [Marshmallow and Raspberry flavors]	**Adults and Children over 12 yrs:** 7.5 - 15 mL po hs. **Children 6-12 yrs:** 2.5 - 3.75 mL po hs.
Castor Oil	**Liquid:** (pure)	**Adults and Children over 12 yrs:** 15 - 60 mL po. **Children 6-12 yrs:** 5 - 15 mL po.
Citrate of Magnesia	**Solution:** magnesium citrate	**Adults:** 1 glassful (approximately 240 mL) po. **Children:** 1/2 glassful (approximately 120 mL) po.
COLACE	**Capsules:** docusate sodium (50 mg) **Capsules:** docusate sodium (100 mg) **Syrup (per 5 mL):** docusate sodium (20 mg), alcohol (1%) **Liquid (per mL):** docusate sodium (10 mg)	**Adults and Older Children:** 50 - 200 mg daily po. **Children 6-12 yrs:** 40 - 120 mg daily po. **Children 3-6 yrs:** 20 - 60 mg daily po. **Infants and Children under 3 yrs:** 10 - 40 mg daily po.
CORRECTOL	**Tablets:** yellow phenolphthalein (65 mg), docusate sodium (100 mg)	**Adults and Children over 6 yrs:** 1 or 2 tablets daily po prn, hs or on arising. **Children 6-12 yrs:** 1 tablet daily po prn.
CORRECTOL EXTRA GENTLE	**Tablets:** docusate sodium (100 mg)	**Adults and Children over 12 yrs:** 2 tablets daily po prn. **Children 6-12 yrs:** 1 tablet daily po prn.
DIALOSE	**Tablets:** docusate sodium (100 mg)	**Adults and Children over 12 yrs:** 1 tablets up to tid po. **Children 6-12 yrs:** 1 tablet daily po.
DIALOSE PLUS	**Tablets:** docusate sodium (100 mg), yellow phenolphthalein (65 mg)	**Adults and Children over 12 yrs:** 1 or 2 tablets daily po. **Children 6-12 yrs:** 1 tablet daily po.
DOXIDAN	**Capsules:** yellow phenolphthalein (65 mg), docusate calcium (60 mg)	**Adults and Children over 12 yrs:** 1 or 2 capsules daily po.

TRADE NAME	DOSAGE FORMS and ACTIVE INGREDIENTS	COMMON DOSAGES and ADMINISTRATION
DULCOLAX	**Enteric-Coated Tablets**: bisacodyl (5 mg)	**Adults and Children over 12 yrs**: 2 tablets as a single dose once daily po. **Children 6-12 yrs**: 1 tablet once daily po.
	Suppositories: bisacodyl (10 mg)	**Adults and Children over 12 yrs**: Insert 1 rectally once daily. **Children 6-12 yrs**: Insert 1/2 rectally once daily.
EX-LAX	**Chewable Tablets**: yellow phenolphthalein (90 mg) **Pills**: yellow phenolphthalein (90 mg)	**Adults and Children over 12 yrs**: Chew 1 or 2 tablets (or swallow 1 or 2 pills), preferably hs. **Children 6-12 yrs**: Chew 1/2 tablet (or swallow 1 pill), preferably hs.
EX-LAX, EXTRA GENTLE	**Pills**: yellow phenolphthalein (65 mg), docusate sodium (75 mg)	**Adults and Children over 12 yrs**: 1 or 2 pills po, preferably hs. **Children 6-12 yrs**: 1 pill po, prn.
EX-LAX, MAXIMUM RELIEF	**Pills**: yellow phenolphthalein (135 mg)	**Adults and Children over 12 yrs**: 1 or 2 pills po, preferably hs.
EX-LAX GENTLE NATURE	**Tablets**: sennosides (20 mg)	**Adults and Children over 12 yrs**: 1 or 2 tablets daily po, preferably hs. **Children 6-12 yrs**: 1 tablet daily po, prn.
FEEN-A-MINT	**Gum**: yellow phenolphthalein (97.2 mg)	**Adults and Children over 12 yrs**: Chew 1 piece of gum daily.
	Pills: yellow phenolphthalein (65 mg), docusate sodium (100 mg)	**Adults and Children over 12 yrs**: 1 or 2 pills po, preferably hs. **Children 6-12 yrs**: 1 pill po, prn.
FLEET BISACODYL ENEMA	**Suspension (per 30 mL)**: bisacodyl (10 mg)	**Adults and Children over 12 yrs**: 30 mL rectally. **Children 6-12 yrs**: 15 mL rectally.
FLEET ENEMA	**Solution (per 118 mL)**: dibasic sodium phosphate (7 g), monobasic sodium phosphate (19 g)	**Adults and Children over 12 yrs**: Administer 4 fl. oz. rectally. **Children 2-12 yrs**: Administer 2 fl. oz. rectally.

FLEET FLAVORED CASTOR OIL	**Emulsion (per 15 mL)**: castor oil (10 mL)	**Adults and Children over 12 yrs**: 45 mL po, followed by a glass of cool water. **Children 2-12 yrs**: 15 mL po, followed by a glass of cool water.
FLEET PHOSPHO-SODA	**Solution (per 100 mL)**: dibasic sodium phosphate (18 g), monobasic sodium phosphate (48 g)	**Adults and Children over 12 yrs**: 20 mL po, upon arising and at least 30 minutes before a meal or at bedtime. Dilute recommended dosage with one-half glass (4 fl. oz.) of cool water. Drink, then follow with one glass (8 fl. oz.) of cool water. **Children 10-12 yrs**: 10 mL po, upon arising and at least 30 minutes before a meal or at bedtime. Dilute recommended dosage with one-half glass (4 fl. oz.) of cool water. Drink, then follow with one glass (8 fl. oz.) of cool water. **Children 5-9 yrs**: 5 mL po, upon arising and at least 30 minutes before a meal or at bedtime. Dilute recommended dosage with one-half glass (4 fl. oz.) of cool water. Drink, then follow with one glass (8 fl. oz.) of cool water.
HALEY'S M-O	**Suspension (per 5 mL)**: magnesium hydroxide (301 mg), mineral oil (1.25 mL) [Plain and Flavored].	**Adults and Children over 12 yrs**: 15 - 30 mL po hs and upon arising. **Children 6-12 yrs**: 5 - 15 mL po once daily.
KASOF	**Capsules**: docusate potassium (240 mg)	**Adults**: 1 capsule daily po.
NATURE'S REMEDY ENEMA	**Solution (per 118 mL)**: sodium biphosphate (19 g), sodium phosphate (7 g)	**Adults and Children over 12 yrs**: One bottle (118 mL delivered dose) rectally. **Children over 2 yrs**: One-half of the adult dose.
NEOLOID	**Emulsion**: castor oil (36.4%) emulsified in a peppermint flavored base	**Adults**: 30 - 60 mL po. **Children**: Adjust between adult dose and infant dose. **Infants**: 2.5 - 7.5 mL po.
PERI-COLACE	**Syrup (per 15 mL)**: docusate sodium (60 mg), casanthranol (30 mg), alcohol (10%) **Capsules**: docusate sodium (100 mg), casanthranol (30 mg)	**Adults**: 15 - 30 mL (or 1 - 2 capsules) po hs. In severe cases, 30 mL (or 2 capsules) bid may be used. **Children**: 5 - 15 mL po hs.

TRADE NAME	DOSAGE FORMS and ACTIVE INGREDIENTS	COMMON DOSAGES and ADMINISTRATION
PHILLIPS' GELCAPS	**Capsules**: phenolphthalein (90 mg), docusate sodium (83 mg)	**Adults and Children over 12 yrs**: 1 or 2 capsules daily po with a full glass of water.
PHILLIPS' MILK OF MAGNESIA	**Suspension (per 5 mL)**: magnesium hydroxide (400 mg) [Regular, Mint, and Cherry flavors]	**Adults and Children over 12 yrs**: 30 - 60 mL po followed by a full glass (8 fl. oz.) of liquid. **Children 6-12 yrs**: 15 - 30 mL po followed by a full glass (8 fl. oz.) of liquid. **Children 2-5 yrs**: 5 - 15 mL po followed by a full glass (8 fl. oz.) of liquid.
	Chewable Tablets: magnesium hydroxide (311 mg)	**Adults and Children over 12 yrs**: Chew thoroughly 6 - 8 tablets, preferably before bedtime and follow with a full glass (8 fl. oz.) of liquid. **Children 6-12 yrs**: Chew thoroughly 3 - 4 tablets, preferably before bedtime and follow with a full glass (8 fl. oz.) of liquid. **Children 2-6 yrs**: Chew thoroughly 1 - 2 tablets, preferably before bedtime and follow with a full glass (8 fl. oz.) of liquid.
	Concentrate (per 5 mL): magnesium hydroxide (800 mg) [Strawberry Creme and Orange Vanilla Creme flavors]	**Adults and Children over 12 yrs**: 15 - 30 mL po followed by a full glass (8 fl. oz.) of liquid. **Children 6-12 yrs**: 7.5 - 15 mL po followed by a full glass (8 fl. oz.) of liquid. **Children 2-5 yrs**: 2.5 - 7.5 mL po followed by a full glass (8 fl. oz.) of liquid.
PURGE	**Liquid**: castor oil (95%) in a sweetened lemon flavored base	**Adults**: 30 - 60 mL po. **Children**: Adjust between adult dose and infant dose. **Infants**: 5 - 10 mL po.

SENOKOT	**Syrup (per 5 mL)**: sennosides (8.8 mg) **Tablets**: sennosides (8.6 mg)	**Adults and Children over 12 yrs**: 10 mL (or 2 tablets) once daily po, preferably hs. Maximum dosage: 20 mL (or 4 tablets) bid po. **Children 6-12 yrs**: 5 mL (or 1 tablet) once daily po, preferably hs. Maximum dosage: 10 mL (or 2 tablets) bid po. **Children 2-6 yrs**: 2.5 mL (or 1/2 tablet) once daily po, preferably hs. Maximum dosage: 5 mL (or 1 tablet) bid po.
	Granules: sennosides (15 mg) per teaspoonful	**Adults and Children over 12 yrs**: 1 teaspoonful once daily po, preferably hs. Maximum dosage: 2 teaspoonfuls bid po. **Children 6-12 yrs**: 1/2 teaspoonful once daily po, preferably hs. Maximum dosage: 1 teaspoonful bid po. **Children 2-6 yrs**: 1/4 teaspoonful once daily po, preferably hs. Maximum dosage: 1/2 teaspoonful bid po.
	Suppositories: senna concentrate (652 mg)	**Adults and Children over 12 yrs**: Insert 1 suppository rectally hs. **Children 6-12 yrs (over 60 lbs)**: Insert 1/2 suppository rectally hs.
SENOKOT-S	**Tablets**: sennosides (8.6 mg), docusate sodium (50 mg)	**Adults and Children over 12 yrs**: 2 tablets once daily po, preferably hs. Maximum dosage: 4 tablets bid po. **Children 6-12 yrs**: 1 tablet once daily po, preferably hs. Maximum dosage: 2 tablets bid po. **Children 2-6 yrs**: 1/2 tablet once daily po, preferably hs. Maximum dosage: 1 tablet bid po.
SENOKOTXTRA	**Tablets**: sennosides (17.2 mg)	**Adults and Children over 12 yrs**: 1 tablet once daily po, preferably hs. Maximum dosage: 2 tablets bid po. **Children 2-6 yrs**: 1/2 tablet once daily po, preferably hs. Maximum dosage: 1 tablet bid po.
SURFAK	**Capsules**: docusate calcium (240 mg)	**Adults and Children over 12 yrs**: 1 capsule daily po.

TABLE Q. DRUGS POTENTIALLY USEFUL IN MANAGING GASTROINTESTINAL PROBLEMS WITH NSAIDS

TRADE NAME	THERAPEUTIC CATEGORY	DOSAGE FORMS AND ACTIVE INGREDIENTS	COMMON ADULT DOSAGE
ALTERNAGEL	Antacid[1, 2]	**Liq (per 5 mL)**: dried aluminum hydroxide gel (600 mg) [Acid Neutralizing Capacity: 16 mEq; Sodium: less than 2.5 mg (0.109 mEq)]	**Hyperacidity**: 5 - 10 mL po prn, between meals and hs. Do not exceed 90 mL in 24 h.
ALU-CAP	Antacid[1, 2]	**Cpsl**: dried aluminum hydroxide gel (equivalent to 400 mg of aluminum hydroxide)	**Hyperacidity**: 3 capsules tid po.
ALUDROX	Antacid[1, 2]	**Susp (per 5 mL)**: aluminum hydroxide gel (307 mg), magnesium hydroxide (103 mg) [Acid Neutralizing Capacity: 12 mEq; Sodium: 0.1 mEq]	**Hyperacidity**: 10 mL q 4 h. Do not exceed 60 mL in 24 h.
ALU-TAB	Antacid[1, 2]	**Tab**: dried aluminum hydroxide gel (equivalent to 500 mg of aluminum hydroxide)	**Hyperacidity**: 3 tablets tid po.
AMPHOJEL	Antacid[1, 2]	**Susp (per 5 mL)**: aluminum hydroxide gel (320 mg) [Acid Neutralizing Capacity: 10 mEq; Sodium: not more than 0.1 mEq]	**Hyperacidity**: 10 mL 5 or 6 times daily po, between meals and hs. Do not exceed 60 mL in 24 h.
		Tab: aluminum hydroxide gel (300 mg) [Acid Neutralizing Capacity: 8 mEq; Sodium: 0.08 mEq]	**Hyperacidity**: 2 tablets 5 or 6 times daily po, between meals and hs. Do not exceed 12 tablets in 24 h.
		Tab: aluminum hydroxide gel (600 mg) [Acid Neutralizing Capacity: 8 mEq; Sodium: 0.13 mEq]	**Hyperacidity**: 1 tablet 5 or 6 times daily po, between meals and hs. Do not exceed 6 tablets in 24 h.

AXID	Histamine H_2-Receptor Blocker[1]	**Cpsl**: nizatidine (150 or 300 mg)	**Active Duodenal Ulcer**: 300 mg once daily po hs or 150 mg bid po. **Maintenance of Healed Duodenal Ulcer**: 150 mg once daily po hs. **Gastroesophageal Reflux Disease**: 150 mg bid po.
BASALJEL	Antacid[1, 2]	**Susp (per 5 mL)**: basic aluminum carbonate gel (equivalent to 400 mg of aluminum hydroxide) [Acid Neutralizing Capacity: 12.5 mEq; Sodium: 0.13 mEq] **Cpsl**: basic aluminum carbonate gel (equivalent to 608 mg of aluminum hydroxide) [Acid Neutralizing Capacity: 12 mEq; Sodium: 0.12 mEq] **Tab**: basic aluminum carbonate gel (equivalent to 608 mg of aluminum hydroxide) [Acid Neutralizing Capacity: 12 mEq; Sodium: 0.12 mEq]	**Hyperacidity**: 10 mL in water or fruit juice, as often as q 2 h po up to 12 times daily. Do not exceed 120 mL in 24 h. **Hyperacidity**: 2 capsules as often as q 2 h po up to 12 times daily. Do not exceed 24 capsules in 24 h. **Hyperacidity**: 2 tablets as often as q 2 h po up to 12 times daily. Do not exceed 24 tablets in 24 h.
CARAFATE	Anti-Ulcer Agent[1]	**Tab**: sucralfate (1 g)	**Active Duodenal Ulcer**: 1 g qid po on an empty stomach. **Maintenance**: 1 g bid po.
CYTOTEC	Anti-Ulcer Agent	**Tab**: misoprostol (100 or 200 μg)	**Prevention of NSAID-induced Gastric Ulcers**: 200 μg qid with food po.
GAVISCON	Antacid[1, 2]	**Liq (per 15 mL)**: aluminum hydroxide (95 mg), magnesium carbonate (358 mg) [Sodium: 1.7 mEq] **Chewable Tab**: dried aluminum hydroxide gel (80 mg), magnesium trisilicate (20 mg) [Sodium: 0.8 mEq]	**Hyperacidity**: 15 - 30 mL qid po, pc and hs, followed by half a glass of water. Do not exceed 120 mL in 24 h. **Hyperacidity**: Chew 2 - 4 tablets qid, pc and hs or prn. Follow each dose with half glass of water or other liquid. Do not exceed 16 tablets in 24 h.

TRADE NAME	THERAPEUTIC CATEGORY	DOSAGE FORMS AND ACTIVE INGREDIENTS	COMMON ADULT DOSAGE
GAVISCON EXTRA STRENGTH RELIEF FORMULA	Antacid[1, 2]	**Liq (per 10 mL)**: aluminum hydroxide (508 mg), magnesium carbonate (475 mg) [Sodium: 1.8 mEq]	**Hyperacidity**: 10 - 20 mL qid po, pc and hs, followed by half a glass of water. Do not exceed 80 mL in 24 hours.
		Chewable Tab: aluminum hydroxide (160 mg), magnesium carbonate (105 mg) [Sodium: 1.3 mEq]	**Hyperacidity**: Chew 2 - 4 tablets qid, pc and hs or prn. Follow each dose with half a glass of water or other liquid. Do not exceed 16 tablets in 24 h.
GAVISCON-2	Antacid[1, 2]	**Chewable Tab**: dried aluminum hydroxide gel (160 mg), magnesium trisilicate (40 mg) [Sodium: 1.6 mEq]	**Hyperacidity**: Chew 1 - 2 tablets qid, pc and hs or prn. Follow each dose with half glass of water or other liquid. Do not exceed 8 tablets in 24 h.
MAALOX	Antacid[1, 2]	**Susp (per 5 mL)**: aluminum hydroxide (225 mg), magnesium hydroxide (200 mg) [Mint and Cherry Creme flavors]. [Acid Neutralizing Capacity: 13.3 mEq; Sodium: 0.06 mg]	**Hyperacidity**: 10 - 20 mL po, pc and hs. Do not exceed 80 mL in 24 h.
		Cplt: calcium carbonate (1000 mg) [Acid Neutralizing Capacity: 20 mEq; Sodium 0.4 mg]	**Hyperacidity**: 1 caplet po prn. Do not exceed 8 caplets in 24 h.
MAALOX HRF	Antacid[1, 2]	**Susp (per 10 mL)**: aluminum hydroxide-magnesium carbonate codried gel (280 mg), magnesium carbonate (350 mg) [Acid Neutralizing Capacity: 9.5 mEq; Sodium: 2 mg]	**Hyperacidity**: 10 - 20 mL po, pc and hs. Do not exceed 80 mL in 24 h.
		Chewable Tab: aluminum hydroxide-magnesium carbonate codried gel (180 mg), magnesium carbonate (160 mg) [Acid Neutralizing Capacity: 7.35 mEq]	**Hyperacidity**: Chew 2 - 4 tablets pc & hs. Follow with 4 fl. oz. of water or other liquid. Do not exceed 16 tablets in 24 h.
MAALOX TC	Antacid[1, 2]	**Susp (per 5 mL)**: aluminum hydroxide (600 mg), magnesium hydroxide (300 mg) [Acid Neutralizing Capacity: 27.2 mEq; Sodium: 0.8 mg (0.03 mEq; dietetically insignificant)]	**Hyperacidity**: 5 - 10 mL qid po, 20 - 60 minutes after meals and hs. Do not exceed 40 mL in 24 h.

MYLANTA GELCAPS	Antacid[1, 2]	**Gelcaps**: calcium carbonate (311 mg), magnesium carbonate (232 mg) [Acid Neutralizing Capacity: 11.5 mEq]	**Hyperacidity**: 2 - 4 gelcaps po prn. Do not take more than 24 gelcaps in 24 h.
PEPCID	Histamine H_2-Receptor Blocker[1]	**Powd for Susp**: famotidine (40 mg/5 mL) **Tab**: famotidine (20 or 40 mg)	**Duodenal Ulcer:** **Acute**: 40 mg hs po; or 20 mg bid po. **Maintenance**: 20 mg hs po. **Active Benign Gastric Ulcer**: 40 mg hs po. **Pathological Hypersecretory Conditions**: 20 mg q 6 h po. **Gastroesophageal Reflux Disease**: 20 mg bid po for up to 6 weeks.
RIOPAN	Antacid[1, 2]	**Susp (per 5 mL)**: magaldrate (540 mg) [Acid Neutralizing Capacity: 15.0 mEq; Sodium: less than 0.013 mEq (considered dietetically sodium free)] **Tab**: magaldrate (480 mg) [Acid Neutralizing Capacity: 13.5 mEq; Sodium: less than 0.004 mEq (considered dietetically sodium free)]	**Hyperacidity**: 5 - 10 mL po between meals and hs. Do not exceed 90 mL in 24 h. **Hyperacidity**: 1 or 2 tablets po between meals and hs. Do not exceed 20 tablets in 24 h.
TAGAMET	Histamine H_2-Receptor Blocker[1]	**Liquid**: cimetidine (300 mg/5 mL) (2.8% alcohol) **Tab**: cimetidine (200, 300, 400 or 800 mg)	**Duodenal Ulcer:** **Active**: 800 mg hs po; or 300 mg qid po with meals & hs; or 400 mg bid po in the AM and PM. **Maintenance**: 400 mg hs po. **Active Benign Gastric Ulcer**: 800 mg hs po; or 300 mg qid po with meals & hs. **Erosive Gastroesophageal Reflux Disease**: 800 mg bid po; or 400 mg qid po for 12 weeks. **Pathological Hypersecretory Conditions**: 300 mg qid po with meals & hs.

TRADE NAME	THERAPEUTIC CATEGORY	DOSAGE FORMS AND ACTIVE INGREDIENTS	COMMON ADULT DOSAGE
ZANTAC	Histamine H_2-Receptor Blocker[1]	**Syrup**: ranitidine HCl (15 mg/mL) (7.5% alcohol) **Tab**: ranitidine HCl (150 or 300 mg)	**Active Duodenal Ulcer**: 150 mg bid po; or 300 mg once daily po hs. **Maintenance Therapy**: 150 mg daily po hs. **Pathological Hypersecretory Conditions**: 150 mg bid po, or more frequently if needed. **Gastroesophageal Reflux and Benign Gastric Ulcer**: 150 mg bid po. **Erosive Esophagitis**: 150 mg qid po.

[1] Not officially indicated for gastrointestinal upset caused by NSAIDs.
[2] Only used as an example of an antacid which can be taken; not a complete listing of antacids available.

INDEX

A

B

C

D

E

F

G

H

I

J

K

L

M

N

O

P

R

S

T

U

V

W

X

Y

Z

Notes

Notes

Notes

Notes

Notes

ORDER FORM FOR HANDBOOKS

TITLE	PRICE x QUANTITY
Handbook on Pain Management, Fourth Edition (1994)	$ 15.00 x ____ = $ ____.___
Handbook of Commonly Prescribed Drugs, Ninth Edition (1994)	$ 15.00 x ____ = $ ____.___
Handbook of Commonly Prescribed Geriatric Drugs, First Edition (1993)	$ 15.00 x ____ = $ ____.___
Handbook of Commonly Prescribed Pediatric Drugs, Fourth Edition (1992)	$ 14.00 x ____ = $ ____.___
Handbook of Common Orthopaedic Fractures, Second Edition (1992)	$ 14.00 x ____ = $ ____.___
Handbook of Commonly Prescribed Ocular Drugs (1991)	$ 13.00 x ____ = $ ____.___
Handbook of Over-the-Counter Preparations (1988)	$ 10.50 x ____ = $ ____.___
	SUB-TOTAL = $ ____.___
Shipping and Handling	= $ 3. 50
PA Residents: Add 6% Sales Tax	= $ ____.___
	TOTAL = $ ____.___

Send mail orders for Handbooks with checks or money orders to:

MEDICAL SURVEILLANCE INC.
P.O. Box 1629 West Chester, PA 19380

(PLEASE PRINT)

Name______________________________ Degree__________

Organization______________________________

Street Address______________________________

City______________________ State______ Zip__________

Telephone Number______________________________

Signature______________________________

FOR FURTHER INFORMATION CALL COLLECT: 610 - 436-8881
FAX: 610 - 436-1803

ORDER FORM FOR COMPUTER DATABASE

TITLE	PRICE x QUANTITY
Pediatric, Adult and Geriatric DrugBase 1.0 (1993)*	$ 49.95 x ____ = $ _____.__
	SUB-TOTAL = $ _____.__
Shipping and Handling	= $ 4.50
PA Residents: Add 6% Sales Tax	= $ _____.__
	TOTAL = $ _____.__

* **System Requirements**: To use Pediatric, Adult and Geriatric DrugBase 1.0, you must have an IBM or IBM compatible XT, AT or PS/2 computer (minimum 512 Kb of RAM memory) and the program must be installed on a hard drive (minimum of 5.5 Mb of free hard disk space). The software may be run with any version of DOS above 2.0; however, DOS 3.0 or higher is recommended.

The DrugBase 1.0 is fully compatible with Microsoft Windows and other multi-tasking software (e.g., Software Carousel). With such software the user can run the DrugBase concurrently with other software applications (such as patient database and prescription writing software) and can quickly switch between the applications.

Annual DrugBase updates will be offered at a reduced price of $ 30.00 per year to buyers for two (2) consecutive years after the purchase of the program.

Send mail orders for the DataBase with checks or money orders to:

MEDICAL SURVEILLANCE INC.
P.O. Box 1629 West Chester, PA 19380

(PLEASE PRINT)

Name____Degree_____________

Organization____

Street Address____

City____State______Zip__________

Telephone Number____

Signature____

FOR FURTHER INFORMATION CALL COLLECT: 610 - 436-8881
FAX: 610 - 436-1803

REQUEST FOR INFORMATION

If you wish to be placed on the mailing list for information concerning new publications and updates, please fill out the form below and mail to:

MEDICAL SURVEILLANCE INC.
P.O. Box 1629 West Chester, PA 19380

(PLEASE PRINT)

Name____

Organization______________________________________

Street Address_____________________________________

City___________________________________State_______

Zip Code_______________

Telephone Number (Optional)____________________________

FOR FURTHER INFORMATION CALL: 610 - 436-8881